The Nursing Associate
at a Glance

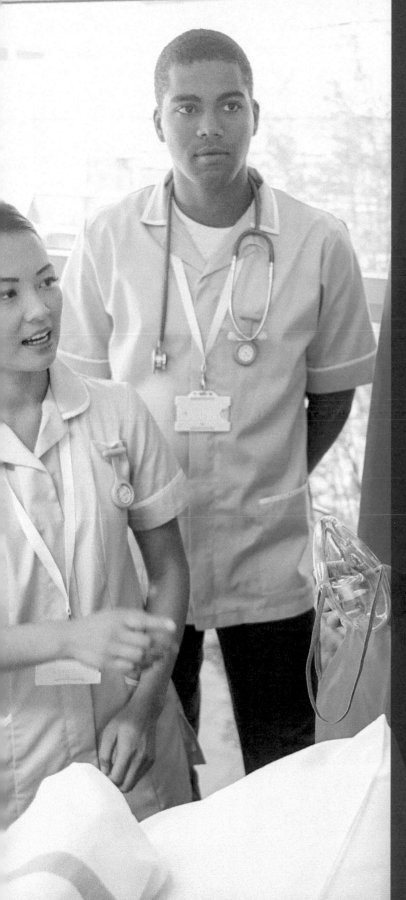

The Nursing Associate
at a Glance

Ian Peate OBE FRCN
Principal, School of Health Studies
Gibraltar Health Authority
Gibraltar

WILEY Blackwell

Registered Office(s)
John Wiley & Sons, Inc., 111 River Street, Hoboken, NJ 07030, USA
John Wiley & Sons Ltd, The Atrium, Southern Gate, Chichester, West Sussex, PO19 8SQ, UK

Editorial Office
9600 Garsington Road, Oxford, OX4 2DQ, UK

For details of our global editorial offices, customer services, and more information about Wiley products, visit us at www.wiley.com.

Wiley also publishes its books in a variety of electronic formats and by print-on-demand. Some content that appears in standard print versions of this book may not be available in other formats.

Library of Congress Cataloging-in-Publication Data

Names: Peate, Ian, author.
Title: The nursing associate at a glance / Ian Peate.
Other titles: At a glance series (Oxford, England)
Description: Hoboken, NJ : Wiley-Blackwell, 2021. | Series: At a glance
    series | Includes bibliographical references and index.
Identifiers: LCCN 2021008652 (print) | LCCN 2021008653 (ebook) |
    ISBN 9781119724308 (paperback) | ISBN 9781119724360 (adobe pdf) |
    ISBN 9781119724353 (epub)
Subjects: MESH: Nursing Assistants | Nursing Care–methods | Nurse's Role |
    United Kingdom | Handbook
Classification: LCC RT41 (print) | LCC RT41 (ebook) | NLM WY 49 | DDC
    610.73–dc23
LC record available at https://lccn.loc.gov/2021008652
LC ebook record available at https://lccn.loc.gov/2021008653

Cover Design: Wiley
Cover Image: © sturti/iStock/Getty Images

Set in 9.5/11.5pt Minion Pro by SPi Global, Pondicherry, India
Printed and bound by CPI Group (UK) Ltd, Croydon, CR0 4YY

C9781119724308_060421

Contents

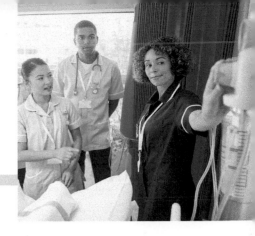

Working in teams 101

Improving safety and quality of care 117

Contributing to integrated care 133

Preface

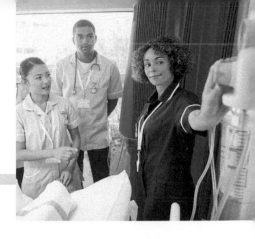

Nursing, being a practice-based discipline, requires the theoretical knowledge provided to be grounded in practice so as to facilitate professional competence with regard to fitness for practice, purpose, award as well as professional standing.

The role of the Nursing Associate was developed in response to a number of key policies and drivers, including the NHS Five Year Forward Plan (NHS, 2014), Shape of Caring: Raising the Bar (Health Education England (HEE) 2015), Nursing Associate Curriculum Framework (HEE, 2017) and the Skills for Health (2017) Nursing Associate Apprenticeship Standards. The Nursing and Midwifery Council (NMC) confirmed in January 2017 that the Nursing Associate will be a new regulated nursing role, in England, from January 2019.

In response to the NMC's confirmation that it would become the Nursing Associate regulator, actions needed to be taken to ensure that standards were in place. Standards were produced in 2018 for the Nursing Associate proficiencies (NMC, 2018a) and for Nursing Associate programmes (NMC, 2018b). The NMC revised its Code of Conduct in 2018 to include the Nursing Associate (NMC, 2018c).

Locally, nationally and globally, health and care settings are experiencing complex challenges. There has been an increased demand on services with the imperative that patients receive the right care, at the right time and in the right place. Key to this is the building of new health and care partnerships, integrating care provision and developing new roles. The Nursing Associate role is a response to the need to develop the healthcare support worker role and to offer support to the Registered Nurse. A role in its own right, the Nursing Associate acts as a bridge between, and complements, the unregulated healthcare workforce and the Registered Nurse. Furthermore, it widens access to further career development as a Registered Nurse.

Approved Nursing Associate programmes are aimed at individuals who are employed in health and care settings. Programmes of study have to be flexible, authentic work-based learning programmes that develop competent, confident and compassionate Nursing Associates who will be proficient in the provision of high-quality, safe and responsive person-centred care that traverses the lifespan in a variety of diverse settings. As programmes of study involve learning *from practice*, and learning *in practice*, they draw upon the principles of work-based learning in supportive environments.

The aim of the Nursing Associate programme should be that on completion of their programme the Trainee Nursing Associate will demonstrate passion and confidence in their practice, committed to supporting the holistic delivery of person-centred care across the life span, embracing the notion of lifelong learning and taking on responsibility for working within their scope of practice.

The six platforms used by the NMC in the Standards of Proficiency for Nursing Associates (NMC, 2018a) have been used to structure the text. Annexes A and B are provided as appendices.

The Nursing Associate at a Glance provides the Trainee Nursing Associate with a revision aid that will support their classroom and practice-based learning. The text aims to help develop Nursing Associates who are competent, confident and compassionate, providing high-quality, evidence-based, holistic, non-judgemental person-centred care.

Terminology

The words that are used to describe people are important. The importance of the terms chosen is that they have the potential to create a particular perception of a person that could be positive, encouraging, enriching or destructive and stigmatising.

Alternatives to the term 'patient' like 'clients', 'service users' and 'consumers' have arisen as a consequence of attempts to empower patients by transforming their relationships with illness, society and health and social care professions. Where 'patients' is used in this text, this also means those people who are in your care and would include service users. In contemporary health and social care, patients are justifiably seen as experts who have valuable lessons to teach practitioners. It should be noted that any form of labelling will always have the potential to do harm.

References

Health Education England (HEE) (2015). Shape of caring: Raising the bar. https://www.hee.nhs.uk/sites/default/files/documents/2348-Shape-of-caring-review-FINAL.pdf. Last accessed August 2020.

Health Education England (HEE) (2017). Nursing Associate Curriculum Framework. https://www.hee.nhs.uk/sites/default/files/documents/Nursing%20Associate%20Curriculum%20Framework%20Feb2017_0.pdf. Last accessed August 2020.

NHS (2014). Five Year Forward Plan. https://www.england.nhs.uk/wp-content/uploads/2014/10/5yfv-web.pdf. Last accessed August 2020.

Nursing and Midwifery Council (NMC) (2018a). Standards of proficiency for nursing associates. https://www.nmc.org.uk/standards/standards-for-nursing-associates/standards-of-proficiency-for-nursing-associates/ Last accessed August 2020.

Nursing and Midwifery Council (NMC) (2018b). Standards for pre-registration nursing associate programmes. https://www.nmc.org.uk/standards/standards-for-nursing-associates/standards-for-pre-registration-nursing-associate-programmes/ Last accessed August 2020.

Nursing and Midwifery Council (NMC) (2018c). The Code. Professional standards of practice and behaviour for nurses, midwives and nursing associates. https://www.nmc.org.uk/globalassets/sitedocuments/nmc-publications/nmc-code.pdf. Last accessed August 2020.

Skills for Health (2017). Nursing Associate Apprenticeship Standards. https://haso.skillsforhealth.org.uk/wp-content/uploads/2017/04/2018.01.12-L5-Nursing-Associate-ST0508-Standard.pdf. Last accessed August 2020.

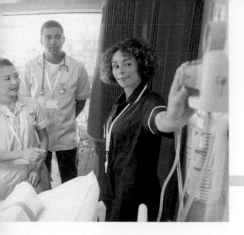

Acknowledgements

I would like to thank my partner, Jussi Lahtinen, for his support and encouragement.

I am grateful to all of the Trainee Nursing Associates and Nursing Associates who inspire and motivate me.

Being an accountable practitioner

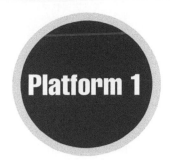

Platform 1

Chapters

1 The Code

At the point of registration, the Nursing Associate will be able to: understand and act in accordance with the Code – professional standards of practice and behaviour for nurses, midwives and Nursing Associates – and fulfil all registration requirements.

Figure 1.1 The Code.

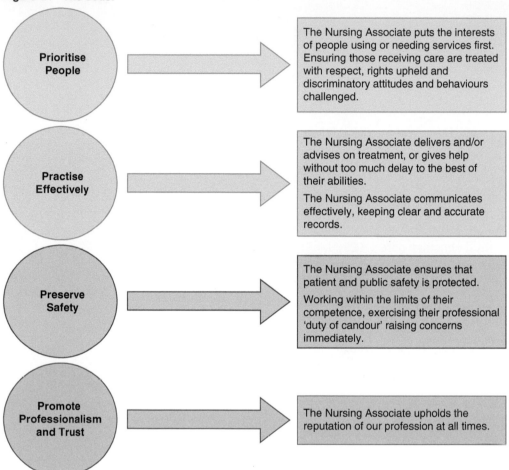

Prioritise People → The Nursing Associate puts the interests of people using or needing services first. Ensuring those receiving care are treated with respect, rights upheld and discriminatory attitudes and behaviours challenged.

Practise Effectively → The Nursing Associate delivers and/or advises on treatment, or gives help without too much delay to the best of their abilities.

The Nursing Associate communicates effectively, keeping clear and accurate records.

Preserve Safety → The Nursing Associate ensures that patient and public safety is protected.

Working within the limits of their competence, exercising their professional 'duty of candour' raising concerns immediately.

Promote Professionalism and Trust → The Nursing Associate upholds the reputation of our profession at all times.

Top Tip

The standards within the Code are what the Nursing Associate commits to when joining or renewing their registration with the Nursing and Midwifery Council (NMC). The professional standards of practice and behaviour are fundamental to being a part of the nursing profession.

The Nursing Associate at a Glance, First Edition. Ian Peate.
© 2021 John Wiley & Sons Ltd. Published 2021 by John Wiley & Sons Ltd.

The Code

The Nursing and Midwifery Council (NMC) functions so as to protect the public. They do this is in a number of ways, for example, by ensuring that only those who meet their requirements are permitted to practise as a nurse or midwife in the UK, or in England, as a Nursing Associate. The NMC will take action if there are any concerns raised about whether a Nursing Associate is fit to practise. In serious cases, this action can lead to the Nursing Associate's name being removed from the professional register.

The NMC (2018) publishes its Code of Conduct (The Code. Professional Standards of Practice and Behaviours for Nurses, Midwives and Nursing Associates) setting out common standards of conduct and behaviour for those on the register. This aim of the Code is to provide a clear, consistent and positive message to others including patients, service users and colleagues about what it is that they can expect from the Nursing Associate who provides nursing care. The Code describes the professional standards that Nursing Associates must uphold.

Nursing Associates must act in line with the Code, irrespective of whether they are providing direct care to individual people, groups or communities or they are drawing on their professional knowledge to influence nursing practice in other roles, for example, leadership, education or research. The values and principles in the Code are relevant in a range of practice settings; they are not, however, negotiable or optional.

There are four key themes in the Code (see Figure 1.1). The Code applies to all Nursing Associates regardless of where they are practising, for example, in primary care, community, acute care, with adults, older people, children and young people or in places of detention. The Code is generic in nature in so far as it not applicable to any one specific field of nursing, it pertains to learning disabilities nursing, children and young people's nursing, mental health nursing and adult nursing and across the lifespan. The Nursing Associate may also be working in a social care setting, criminal justice setting, with the homeless, working with families and other agencies; regardless, the Code applies.

Prioritise people

At all times the Nursing Associate is required to ensure that the interests of people using or needing nursing services will come first. The care and safety of people are the Nursing Associate's key concerns; dignity is to be preserved, and needs are to be acknowledged, assessed and responded to. Those who receive care are to be treated with respect, their rights upheld and discriminatory attitudes and behaviours challenged.

Practise effectively

Care delivery or the provision of advice on treatment or providing help (including preventative or rehabilitative care) must be done without too much delay, to the best of abilities. Care is provided on the basis of the best evidence available and best practice. The Nursing Associate must communicate effectively, maintain clear and accurate records and share skills, knowledge and experience where appropriate. They must reflect and act on any feedback received so as to improve their practice.

Preserve safety

When practising, the Nursing Associate must ensure that patient and public safety is not affected, working within the limits of their competence. Exercise the professional 'duty of candour' and raise concerns without delay whenever there are situations that put patients or public safety at risk. Where appropriate take necessary action to deal with any concerns.

Promote professionalism and trust

The reputation of the profession must be upheld at all times, and the Nursing Associate is required to display a personal commitment to the standards of practice and behaviour set out in the Code. The Nursing Associate should be a model of integrity and leadership that others would wish to aspire to. This should lead to trust and confidence in the profession from patients, people receiving care, other health and care professionals as well as the public.

The NMC provides a framework against which the Nursing Associate practises. The Nursing Associate's primary duty is to the people whom they care and offer support to; actions (or omissions) will be judged against the backdrop of the Code. Nursing Associate is a protected title and may only be used by someone on the NMC's register.

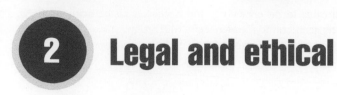

2 Legal and ethical

At the point of registration, the Nursing Associate will be able to: understand and apply relevant legal, regulatory and governance requirements, policies, and ethical frameworks, including any mandatory reporting duties, to all areas of practice.

Figure 2.1 The law and ethics.

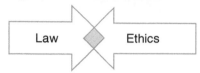

Figure 2.2 Ethics.

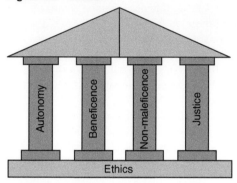

Table 2.1 Governance.

Clinical governance addresses activities that can help to maintain and improve high standards of patient care.	
Policies	National policies have a major impact on the resourcing of services; they also set performance indicators and evaluation criteria. Policies exist that define and integrate appropriate standards for delivery of care, addressing conditions necessary for that care to occur.
Protocols	A document developed to guide decision-making around specific issues. Protocols exist for a wide range of activities. These can range from clinical issues such as caring for someone with an infection through to the procedures required to provide nurse-led physical exercise intervention for people with dementia.
Standards	These reflect a desired and achievable level of performance against which a Nursing Associate's actual performance can be compared. The key aim/purpose is to direct and maintain safe and clinically competent nursing practice.
Guidance	Guidelines are evidence-based recommendations for health and care. They set out the care and services suitable for most people with a specific condition or need and for people in particular circumstances or settings.
Procedures	Using an evidence base. These detail how to do things, for example, the principles of hand hygiene and the procedure for cleaning the hands.

Top Tip

With regard to policies, protocols, standards, guidance and procedures – know them, read them, use them.

The Nursing Associate at a Glance, First Edition. Ian Peate.
© 2021 John Wiley & Sons Ltd. Published 2021 by John Wiley & Sons Ltd.

The law and ethics

The law and ethics permeate every aspect of nursing practice. Often Nursing Associates and others ask the questions 'what is legal' and 'how do I decide what is right' so that I might practise safely and ethically. The law and ethics are intimately related to each other, often overlapping (Figure 2.1). Legal and regulatory frameworks come in the form of law and the Code (NMC, 2018).

Ethics

Ethics can be described as moral philosophy. This is a system of moral principles that are concerned with what is good for individuals and for society. Each interaction the Nursing Associate has with patients involves making a judgement about right or wrong, good or bad. Underpinning each interaction, the principles of patient-centred care are utilised, engaging with the patient at all times. The Nursing Associate needs ask whenever providing care or offering support: is this in the best interests of the patient?

The ethical principles

The four key ethical principles address a value that arises in interactions between healthcare providers and patients. The principles address the issue of being fair, honest and having respect for fellow human beings (see Figure 2.2).

Autonomy

Everybody has the right to control what happens to their bodies (self-determination) based on their values and belief system. Respecting the principle of autonomy means that an adult person who is informed and competent can refuse or accept treatment, drugs and surgery aligned with their wishes. People have the right to control what happens to their bodies because they are free and rational. Decisions made must be respected by everyone, even if those decisions are not in the patient's best interest.

Beneficence

Those who provide health and social care must strive to improve the health of those whom they provide care and support to, to do the most good for the patient in each situation. However, what might be good for one patient may not be good for another, and each situation is considered individually. This principle is about doing good and avoiding malevolence.

Non-maleficence

This principle is the essence of healthcare ethics and is concerned with 'First, do no harm'. At all times the Nursing Associate must avoid causing harm to patients, protecting them from harm.

Justice

The final principle requires the Nursing Associate to be as fair as possible when offering treatment to patients and allocating scarce resources. Access to care should be equitable. At all times the Nursing Associate must be able to justify their actions in each situation.

Law

Law is a system of rules and guidelines enforced through social institutions such as the criminal justice system to govern behaviour. Law plays a key role in the provision of contemporary health and social care. Much legislation has been passed that has a profound effect on how care is delivered, for example, the Children Act, The Mental Health Act, Capacity Act and the Health and Social Care Act.

Parallels with ethics and law

Ethics and law are closely related. Laws are made based on the moral values of society (in general), describing the basic behaviour of people. They represent the minimum standards of human behaviours, that is, ethical behaviour. Laws and ethics are systems that maintain a set of moral values, preventing people from violating them, providing people with guidelines on what they may or may not do in specific situations.

Ethics comes from people's awareness of what is right and what is wrong. The Code, for example, is enshrined in ethics (see Chapter 1). Laws however, are written and approved by governments. Ethics can vary from person to person as different people can have different opinions on a particular issue. Laws describe what is illegal regardless of the different opinions people might have. In general, ethics are not well defined; however, laws are defined and precise.

Governance requirements are usually in the form of policies, protocols, standards, guidance and procedures (see Table 2.1). Clinical governance activities can help to maintain and improve high standards of patient care.

3 Duty of Candour

At the point of registration, the Nursing Associate will be able to: understand the importance of courage and transparency and apply the Duty of Candour, recognising and reporting any situations, behaviours or errors that could result in poor care outcomes.

Figure 3.1 The duty of candour.

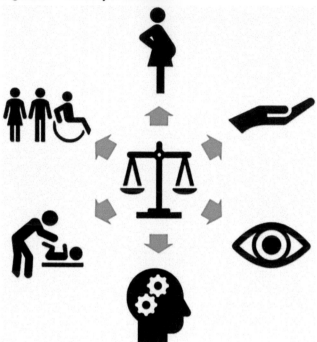

Box 3.1 Six criteria laid out in law that have to be met for a whistleblowing concern.

1 The person raising the concern is a 'worker' (includes employees, agency workers, trainees, volunteers, trainee Nursing Associates, student nurses and student midwives).
2 The person raising the concern must believe they are acting in the public interest.
3 The person raising the concern must believe that it shows past, present or likely future wrongdoing.
4 The person raising the concern must believe that the matter falls within a regulatory remit.
5 The person raising the concern must believe that the information they disclose is true.
6 In raising the concern, the individual must not themselves be committing an offence.

Table 3.1 The 6Cs.

Courage	Being courageous enables the Nursing Associate to do the right thing for the people we care for, to speak up when there are concerns and to respect the Duty of Candour.
Communication	Central to successful caring relationships is communication, caring relationships and effective teamwork.
Commitment	The foundation of successful caring relationships is commitment to patients and communities.
Competence	Being competent means that the Nursing Associate must have the ability to understand an individual's health and social needs.
Compassion	Compassion can be explained as intelligent kindness and is central to how people perceive their care.
Care	Caring defines the Nursing Associate. Those receiving care expect it to be right for them throughout every stage of their life.

Top Tip

The Duty of Candour is the legal duty to be open and honest when things go wrong. The Nursing Associate has a statutory and professional duty to be open and candid with patients about any errors in their care and treatment.

The Nursing Associate at a Glance, First Edition. Ian Peate.
© 2021 John Wiley & Sons Ltd. Published 2021 by John Wiley & Sons Ltd.

The Duty of Candour

Any culture of secrecy or cover-up in healthcare must be challenged. This has led to a focus on making candour in healthcare mandatory. The definition of Candour by the Professional Standards Authority means being honest when something goes wrong. When health and care systems are open, transparent and honest, there are many benefits for the care and treatment of people. The Nursing Associate has a professional duty of candour under the Code, and a statutory duty applies to organisations also. When organisations fail to adhere to this duty, they run the risk of criminal sanctions. One aspect of the duty is to report back to the patient or relatives if there has been any unintended or unexpected incident that could result in, or appears to have resulted in the death of the patient or severe harm, moderate harm or prolonged psychological harm to the patient; these are known as notifiable safety incidents. The duty of candour is all encompassing and impacts widely (Figure 3.1).

The Nursing Associate

The Nursing Associate must be open and honest with patients when something has gone wrong with their treatment or care, or if it has the potential to cause, harm or distress. This means that the patient (or advocate, carer or family, where appropriate) must be told when something has gone wrong, an apology must be given to the patient (or, where appropriate, the patient's advocate, carer or family), if possible an appropriate remedy or support offered to put things right. When an apology is made this does not mean that the practitioner is accepting legal liability for what has occurred, nor that the practitioner is accepting any personal responsibility for the mistakes of others or for systemic failings. The patient must be offered a full explanation of the short and long term effects of what has happened.

As well as being open and honest with patients, the Nursing Associate has to be open and honest with their colleagues, employers and appropriate organisations as well assisting with and taking part in any reviews and investigations when asked. There is also a requirement to be open and honest with the NMC, raising any concerns where appropriate and not preventing someone from raising concerns.

Openness and Honesty

As a Nursing Associate, the Code requires that you are open and honest with patients, colleagues and your employer. The obligation to be open and honest, the professional duty of candour, can sometimes be difficult for Nursing Associates and other health and social care professionals to do for a variety of reasons, nevertheless there is an expectation that they be candid. It is unacceptable that health and social professionals do not tell the truth when a patient has been harmed, be this by withholding or misrepresenting the facts.

Whistleblowing

Whistleblowing is when an individual reports workplace concerns about unsafe care or wrongdoing, it is not the same as a Duty of Candour but, there is an overlap. The law sets out several criteria that must be met for raising concerns to qualify as whistleblowing (see Box 3.1).

If all of the conditions in Box 3.1 are met, the person blowing the whistle enjoys legal protection to prevent them suffering any retaliation from their employer because of what they have done.

Challenges to the Duty of Candour

The workplace culture in which a Nursing Associate practises can influence candour towards patients. Environments that have an ethos of openness are more conducive to being open and honest with patients. Organisations where a blame culture, or a culture of defensiveness exist, are not environments in which the professional duty of candour will thrive.

Courage

Whilst achieving zero harm, is aspirational, it may, in reality be unachievable. Given that proposition, what needs to be put in place is to improve the responses made when harm occurs. Robust governance that would include incident reporting, audit, development of protocols and multidisciplinary education must be seen as central to any change in cultural.

The Duty of Candour requires moral courage, integrity, resilience and support. Courage is one of the 6Cs (see Table 3.1).

Non-discriminatory behaviour

At the point of registration, the Nursing Associate will be able to: demonstrate an understanding of, and the ability to, challenge or report discriminatory behaviour.

Figure 4.1 The nine protected characteristics.

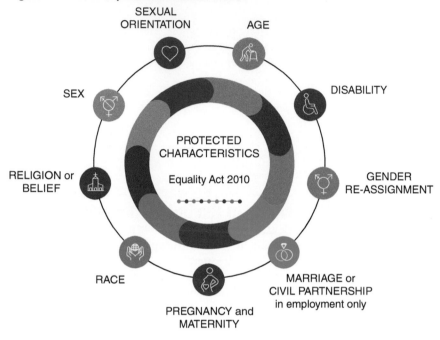

Table 4.1 Types of discrimination.

Type of discrimination	Discussion
Direct discrimination	When a person with a protected characteristic is treated less favourably than others.
Indirect discrimination	If there is a rule, policy or protocol that puts a person at a disadvantage as compared to others, it may be considered indirect discrimination.
Discrimination by association	If a person is treated unfairly because someone you know or are caring for has a protected characteristic, this may be construed as discrimination by association. For example, you are refused service in a restaurant because the person you are with has a disability.
Discrimination by perception	Receiving unfair treatment because someone thinks the person belongs to a group with protected characteristics may be discrimination by perception. For example, a person with a mental health problem is refused a lease for a flat by an estate agent because they assume people with mental health issues behave in a certain way.
Harassment	This comprises unwanted behaviour making another person feel offended, humiliated or intimidated. Unwanted behaviour could include physical gestures, abuse, jokes, spoken or written words or offensive emails and expressions.
Victimisation	When a person is treated badly or subjected to disadvantage because they have complained about discrimination or they have supported another victim of discrimination, this could be considered victimisation.

Top Tip

Never ignore or excuse discriminatory behaviour any more than you would ignore someone if they were in pain.

The Nursing Associate at a Glance, First Edition. Ian Peate.
© 2021 John Wiley & Sons Ltd. Published 2021 by John Wiley & Sons Ltd.

Protected characteristics

In October 2010 the Equality Act came into force, providing a single legal framework with clear, streamlined law to help tackle disadvantage and discrimination in a more effective way. The Equality Act 2010 has identified nine protected characteristics (see Figure 4.1).

Because every person has at least some of these characteristics such as age, race or gender, the Act protects every person from being discriminated against. If a person is treated unfavourably because someone thinks that person belongs to a particular group of people with protected characteristics, this is unlawful discrimination.

Discrimination happens when people are treated differently and negatively because assumptions are made about them or a group to which they belong or appear to belong to. Some examples can include:

- Labelling – giving a 'label' to a group of people because of characteristics, e.g. an individual being labelled as 'Asian' based solely on the colour of their skin
- Stereotyping – assuming traits and characteristics of a group of people e.g. all individuals with autism are highly intelligent
- Prejudice – not liking somebody because of the group they belong to, e.g. racism, sexism, homophobia and so on.

Discriminatory behaviour

Discrimination means treating another person unfairly because of who they are or because they have certain characteristics. If a person has been treated differently from other people only because of who they are or because they possess certain characteristics, then they may have been discriminated against, and discriminatory behaviour is illegal. There are several types of discrimination (see Table 4.1).

Challenging discriminatory behaviour

In order to promote a culture of anti-discrimination, any and all discrimination should be challenged as soon as possible and in a way that encourages change. Discrimination must never be accepted, excused or dismissed; it should always be challenged to be sure that the discriminating individual understands that their behaviour is unacceptable, whether it was deliberate or unintentional.

A public authority is an organisation that provides public services. NHS hospitals or social services are public sector organisations. Private organisations or charities which carry out public services or functions are also known as public authorities, such as, a private care home that is funded by a local authority. If a person has experienced discrimination by a public authority, there are several things that can be done.

If there is an allegation that unlawful discrimination has taken place, one option might be to try to sort out the problem informally at first, for example, talking to the people who are alleged to have been discriminatory. It is important to keep a note, a record, of any conversations or meetings that have taken place.

Employers will have agreed ways of working, and this will provide guidance about challenging and reporting acts of discrimination. The Nursing Associate in training must seek support from their supervisor, line manager or training organisation/university. Policy and procedure will be in place, and these must be adhered to.

Speaking up if somebody is being discriminatory lets the person know that their behaviour is unacceptable and can offer the opportunity to educate them about why discrimination is unacceptable.

Reporting discrimination to your supervisor, manager or making a complaint regarding the person discriminating means that the report/complaint must be taken seriously, and it has to be investigated according to policies and the law.

The Nursing Associate is required to act as an advocate for the vulnerable, challenging discriminatory attitudes and behaviour concerning their care; at all times, you must treat people fairly and without discrimination, bullying or harassment.

5 The demands of professional practice

At the point of registration, the Nursing Associate will be able to: understand the demands of professional practice and demonstrate how to recognise signs of vulnerability in themselves or their colleagues and the action required to minimise risks to health.

Case Study 5.1

I thought I would be able to handle it all, but after about eight months as a Nursing Associate I really started to struggle with anxiety, and I came to a point where I felt crushed and overwhelmed.

Oti was a newly qualified Nursing Associate working as a member of an assessment and treatment specialist service providing care for those with mental illnesses, who also have a diagnosis of a learning disability. This was a newly created post. When Oti commenced the job, her manager, a social worker, was less than complimentary about the role of the Nursing Associate, commenting to Oti how she felt being given an enrolled nurse to do a registered nurse's job was not only unfair to her but to the patients also.

Joining the team, Oti was very much left to her devices as she had no preceptor, and few people (if any) understood the role and function of the Nursing Associate. Oti asked if she could, at the next team meeting, give a short presentation regarding the role of the Nursing Associate, bringing with her one of her lecturers from the university to present with her. On three occasions, the presentation was cancelled, and in fact, it never happened.

The service was being reviewed with plans to restructure provision. In the meantime, Oti came to work and was given several 'tasks and duties' that were commensurate with the role of a healthcare assistant. The job Oti came to do every day was far from the Nursing Associate job she had applied for and was successful in getting. After 3 months, Oti made an appointment to see her manager to discuss how she was getting on. The manager asked her to send her an email as she was too busy for a meeting. Oti complied with this. Three more months passed, and things had not changed. Oti was becoming despondent. She spoke with her staff side representative, who suggested a meeting with her manager. In the next three months, Oti had developed a number of niggling illnesses. She had recurrent colds, she had no self-esteem, she felt she was letting people down, she was not sleeping, she was unable to switch off from her work, she dreaded having to go into work, she told her partner it was soul destroying, she found she was making silly mistakes at work such as inputting data incorrectly and on one occasion she had forgotten to make a follow-up appointment for a service user; she felt she was being deskilled. The service user came into the clinic and verbally abused Oti, making physical threats. Oti went to see her GP, who said she was hypertensive, experiencing stress and was vulnerable. She was signed off sick from work.

Oti returned to work to find out the service had been re-organised, and her new manager, also a social worker, conducted a welcome-back-to-work meeting. A preceptor plan was developed, and a preceptor was allocated to help Oti achieve her future aspirations and to outline how she could become a fully integrated team member making a difference to the care of others. Oti and her preceptor meet regularly, and Oti is able to fully utilise her full scope of practice. She began to feel valued and that she was making a difference to the people she offered care and support to, and she is celebrating her achievements. Recently trainee Nursing Associates have been allocated to the clinic, and Oti is seen as a central resource and as a support to those who are on the same programme that she was on.

Top Tip

It is OK to not be OK. Seek help early, do not let anxieties fester and use all of the resources available including managers and staff side support, for example, your trade union or professional body.

The Nursing Associate at a Glance, First Edition. Ian Peate.
© 2021 John Wiley & Sons Ltd. Published 2021 by John Wiley & Sons Ltd.

Vulnerability

The NMC Standards of Proficiency for the Nursing Associate requires you understand the demands of professional practice and to demonstrate how to recognise signs of vulnerability in yourself or colleagues and to understand the action that is required to minimise risks to health.

Studying nursing is particularly hard: it involves trying to balance assignments, attending placements, working shift patterns, having a social life and, importantly, finding time for yourself. When registered, a Nursing Associate experiences other pressures that replace those faced whilst studying. Professional practice makes many demands. Regardless of the site of practice, on a daily basis the Nursing Associate engages with sensitive, intimate relationships, facing threats of violence and verbal abuse, grief and death. In some places of work, the atmosphere is enclosed; there are time pressures; a need to implement professional knowledge; excessive noise or undue quiet; sudden swings from intense to routine tasks; no second chance; unpleasant sights, sounds and smells and tense working relationships. These experiences and difficulties appear to be further exacerbated by a number of organisational issues which are instrumental in the stress process.

When the Nursing Associate is confronted by such events and tasks, it is hardly surprising that they report high levels of stress, and the physical and mental impact on the Nursing Associate can be detrimental to their health and well-being.

Stress

Whilst there is stress in all jobs, in those careers dealing with human health, the importance of this issue becomes more sensitive and critical. Stress-related factors can be considered as a predictor of caring behaviours.

The experience of stress represents a psychological state. It can come about as a result of exposure, or threat of exposure, to the more tangible workplace hazards as well as to the psycho-social hazards of work. Those hazards of work which are associated with the experience of stress can be termed stressors.

When applied directly to nursing, a situation which is typically experienced as stressful is seen to involve work demands which are threatening or which are not well matched to the knowledge, skills and ability to cope of those involved; or work which does not fulfil their needs, especially where those nurses have little control over work and where they receive little support at work or outside of work.

Recognising vulnerability

Occupational stress negatively affects the Nursing Associates' health-related quality of life; it renders the Nursing Associate vulnerable and can influence patient outcomes. Job-related stress can result in loss of compassion for patients and increased incidences of practice errors, and as such is unfavourably associated with the quality of care.

Verbal or physical abuse can have negative psychological effects that persist after the incident.

With regard to physical health, work-related stress is linked with many physical health problems including migraines, musculoskeletal pain, long-term physical illnesses, hypertension, irritable bowel syndrome and duodenal ulcer, and immune and endocrine system illnesses.

Psychiatric morbidity is also associated with occupational stress, at an emotional level. It has been correlated with anxiety, dysthymia, low self-esteem, depression and feelings of inadequacy. See Case Study 5.1, which outlines the experiences of a vulnerable Nursing Associate who struggled at work to cope.

Responding to stress

In responding to stress and the damaging effect it can have on the Nursing Associate and care outcomes, it is essential to acknowledge that stress has the potential to make the Nursing Associate vulnerable to ill health.

The ability to cope with the demands and stress from work may be improved with specific occupational health education and training programmes that enhance knowledge and ability. The approach must address both the individual and the organisation. Facilitation and verbalisation of feelings and experiences, teaching relaxation techniques, conflict solving and positive reappraisal may help with regard to stress response modification and stress coping. Interventions at an institutional and organisational level (employers and universities), including additional managerial support and staff recognition policies, may be helpful in work environments to prevent stress on a primary level. When dealing with stress, knowing where to go for help is also important.

6 Health and well-being: self-care

At the point of registration, the Nursing Associate will be able to: understand the professional responsibility to adopt a healthy lifestyle to maintain the level of personal fitness and well-being required to meet people's needs for mental and physical care.

Figure 6.1   Some components of good health and well-being.

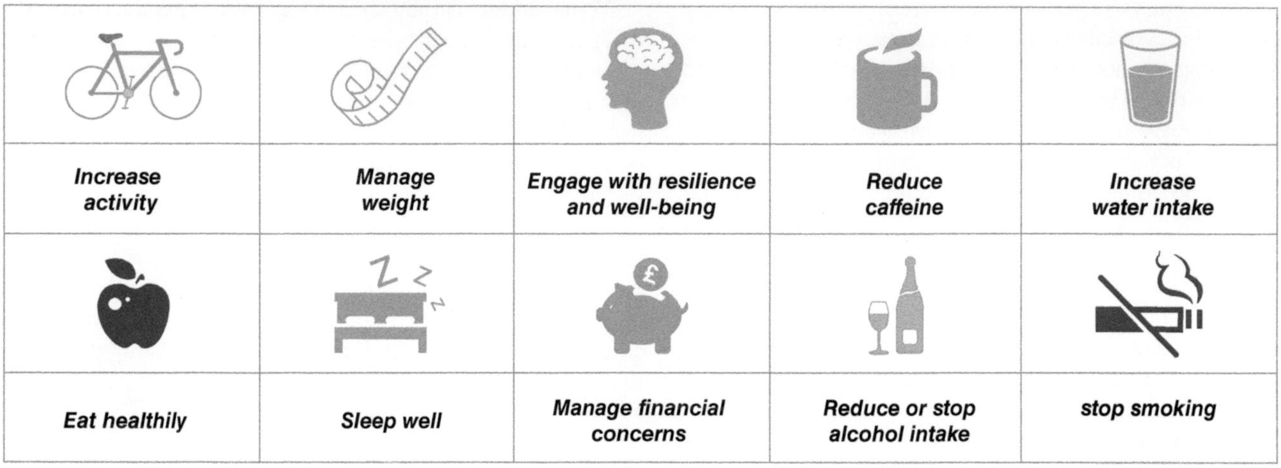

Increase activity	Manage weight	Engage with resilience and well-being	Reduce caffeine	Increase water intake
Eat healthily	Sleep well	Manage financial concerns	Reduce or stop alcohol intake	stop smoking

Top Tip

The Nursing and Midwifery Council's (NMC's) health declaration enables them to determine that those applying to join, renew or be readmitted to the register meet their requirements for health to ensure they can practise safely and effectively.

The Nursing Associate at a Glance, First Edition. Ian Peate.
© 2021 John Wiley & Sons Ltd. Published 2021 by John Wiley & Sons Ltd.

The Nursing and Midwifery Council (NMC)

The health and well-being of any workforce is important. The Nursing Associate needs to look after themselves as well as others. This is also important when they are managing others; the well-being of other staff becomes an added concern. At the point of registration, the NMC Code requires all Nursing Associates to maintain a level of health that permits them to undertake their role effectively as well as engaging in health promotion with patients.

In order to be on the NMC's register, the Nursing Associate must meet a range of professional standards, and one of these concerns is health. Those on the register are part of a profession that has nationally recognised standards that are set by law. When the NMC say that a person is capable of safe and effective practice, they mean that they have the skills, knowledge, character and health to work in their profession safely and effectively.

When an approved programme of study has been successfully completed by the Nursing Associate, this does not guarantee that they will be able to register. Sometimes when a trainee Nursing Associate has completed an education programme and declares information to the NMC, their application may be rejected. All trainee Nursing Associates seeking registration (or once qualified during revalidation) are to be of good health to satisfy the NMC that they are capable of safe and effective practice. The NMC's concern is whether the Nursing Associate has a health condition and/or disability which could affect practice. The NMC needs to be able to assess whether it may place at risk the safety of those they offer care and support to.

The interest in health and well-being over the recent years has gathered momentum significantly with a growing body of evidence that has demonstrated a link with working conditions, support offered by managers and staff engagement with patient outcomes.

Health and well-being

Wellness is so much more than being simply free from illness. 'Health', according to the World Health Organization (2019) is 'a state of complete physical, mental and social well-being and not merely the absence of disease or infirmity'.

The WHO definition explicitly links health with well-being, seeing health as a positive aspiration; health therefore is a means to living well, highlighting the link between health and participation in society, as a human right that requires physical and social resources to achieve and maintain. 'Well-being' refers to a positive rather than neutral state.

Resilience

Resilience is the capacity to bounce back from adversity; sometimes it is also known as emotional resilience. Protective factors increase resilience, and risk factors increase vulnerability. Resilient individuals, families and communities are more able to deal with difficulties and adversities than those with less resilience (University College London 2014). Resilience is associated with the ability to face adverse situations whilst remaining focused, continuing to be optimistic for the future. See also Chapter 8 of this text.

Self-care

The Nursing Associate needs to consider those factors that impact upon their own health; this is sometimes known as self-care. There are several resources available that can help support the Nursing Associate and other nursing staff to take ownership of their own health (physical or/and mental), encouraging them to take the time to apply the same level of care to their own well-being just as they would do for the people they care for and offer support to. The focus needs to on body, mind, heart, work, career, spirit and balance. Figure 6.1 provides an overview of some of the components of healthy living that may lead to enhanced well-being.

The Royal College of Nursing have produced a 'Healthy You Assessment Worksheet'. The self-assessment offers an overview of effective strategies to maintain a healthy you. The lists are not definitive, only suggestions. When completing the assessment, choose one item from each area that you will actively work on to improve.

7 The principles of research and evidence-based practice

At the point of registration, the Nursing Associate will be able to: describe the principles of research and how research findings are used to inform evidence-based practice (EBP).

Figure 7.1 The stages of the nursing research journey. Source: Glasper and Rees (2017).

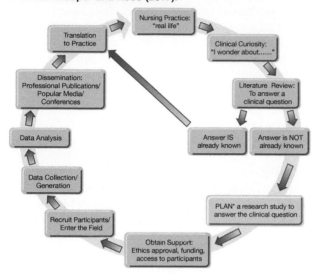

Figure 7.2 Planning: the research process. Source: Glasper and Rees (2017).

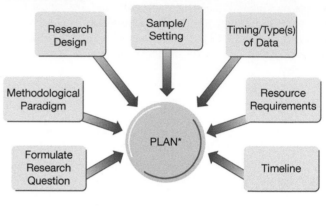

Figure 7.3 Implementation of evidence-based practice (EBP). Source: Glasper and Rees (2017).

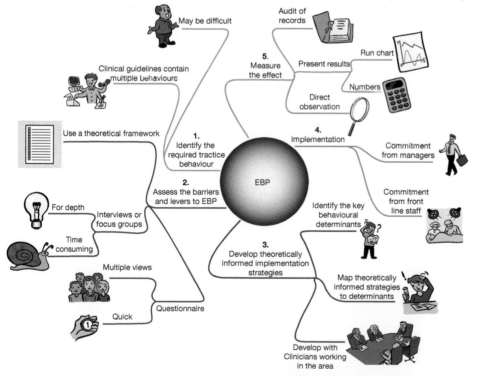

Top Tip

It is not possible to address all aspects of research and evidence-based practice (EBP) in this chapter. Glasper and Rees (2017) have edited an excellent text: *Nursing and Healthcare Research At A Glance*.

The provision of high-quality care is supported by evidence. Gaining knowledge through research and evidence-based practice (EBP) and developing strategies for implementation are key skills for Nursing Associates regardless of the setting.

Research

The purpose of undertaking research is to generate new knowledge or to validate existing knowledge based on a theory. Research studies will involve systematic, scientific inquiry aimed at answering specific research questions or to test hypotheses using analytical, rigorous methods. Although research is about investigation, exploration and discovery, it also requires insight and understanding of the philosophy of science. For research results to be considered reliable and valid, those undertaking the research use the scientific method in orderly, sequential steps. The stages of the nursing research journey can be found in Figure 7.1. The planning stage is depicted in Figure 7.2.

All research is different, and the following principles are common to all good pieces of research involving those using health and social care services, their families and carers and staff:

- A clear statement of research aims, defining the research question.
- Accessible information for participants, explaining what the research is about and what it will involve; consent is obtained in writing on a consent form prior to commencement of research.
- The methodology is appropriate to the research question. Some research use a combination of methodologies, complementing one another.
- The research should be carried out in an unbiased fashion. As far as possible the researcher should not influence the results of the research in any way.
- From the outset, the research should have appropriate and sufficient resources allocated to it.
- Those conducting the research should be trained in research and research methods.

- Those involved in designing, conducting, analysing and supervising the research should have a full understanding of the subject area.
- It may help if the researcher has experience of working in the area.
- If applicable, information generated from the research will inform the policy-making process, and it should be disseminated.
- All research must be ethical and not harmful in any way to participants.

Evidence-based practice

EBP, unlike research, is not concerned with developing new knowledge or validating existing knowledge. EBP is about translating the evidence and then applying this to clinical decision-making situations (see Figure 7.3). One of the overall aims of EBP is to implement the best evidence that is available to make patient-care decisions. Most of the best available evidence is derived from research. EBP, however, goes beyond research use and it also includes clinical expertise as well as patient preferences and values. EBP acknowledges that there are times when the best evidence is that of opinion leaders and experts (and these may include patients), despite the absence of definitive knowledge from research results. Although research is concerned about the development of new knowledge, EBP involves innovation in terms of finding and translating the best evidence into clinical practice.

A number of critical steps are associated with EBP.

The EBP process comprises seven critical steps:

1 Promote a body of inquiry (engender curiosity).
2 Ask a significant clinical question.
3 Collect the most relevant and the best evidence (there are hierarchies of evidence).
4 Critically appraise the evidence (use a systematic approach).
5 Integrate the evidence with clinical expertise, patient preferences and values in making a practice decision or change.
6 Evaluate the practice decision or change.
7 Disseminate EBP results.

8 Emotional intelligence

At the point of registration, the Nursing Associate will be able to: understand and explain the meaning of resilience and emotional intelligence, and their influence on an individual's ability to provide care.

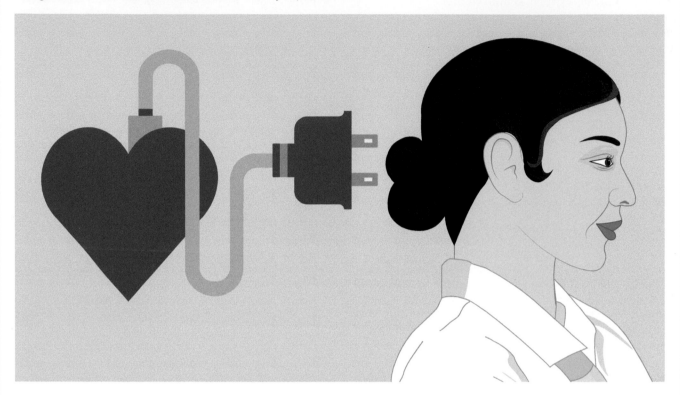

Table 8.1 Four factors of emotional intelligence (Source: Hefferman 2010).

Factor	Description
Well-being	Involves the individual having a good level of self-esteem and the characteristics of feeling happy and satisfied with a positive outlook on life.
Self-control	Is concerned with the ability of the individual to regulate and control their emotional responses, and their competence to handle stress.
Emotionality	Is the skill to show empathy, communicate feelings and be aware of the perspectives of others in a situation
Sociability	Concerns the social competence of the individual, their ability to demonstrate strong social skills and to be assertive and influence others.

Top Tip
Remember, you are only able to provide the best care for others when you are also taking care of yourself.

The Nursing Associate at a Glance, First Edition. Ian Peate.
© 2021 John Wiley & Sons Ltd. Published 2021 by John Wiley & Sons Ltd.

Definition

In 1990 Salovey and Mayer defined emotional intelligence as 'the subset of social intelligence that involves the ability to monitor one's own and others' feelings and emotions, to discriminate among them and to use this information to guide one's thinking and actions'. Those who are emotionally intelligent are able to use, understand as well as manage their feelings in such a way that it can benefit themselves and others.

Emotional intelligence

The concept of emotional intelligence has been identified as being separate from academic intelligence and is required for a person to be successful in the practicalities of life. It is recognised that emotional intelligence is an essential requirement for nursing and other healthcare staff and that some are not aware of this concept or able to identify how they can best manage their own emotions. It is possible for individuals to increase and also further develop their emotional intelligence.

Emotional intelligence includes:

- Feeling but also correctly identifying emotions, both in oneself and in others
- Using these emotions to assist reasoning
- Having the capability to understand feelings
- Managing one's emotions
- Controlling emotional situations.

Development of emotional intelligence can have positive results on several levels. It requires the Nursing Associate to engage in self-reflection and work on oneself; this is not always easy to do. A number of tools are available to assess emotional intelligence. Seeking feedback on behaviour and evaluating how others react to our behaviour can help monitor our own and the feelings and the emotions of others. Using the information gained from feedback helps to guide our thinking and action.

Those who are emotionally intelligent perceive themselves as confident, and they are better able to understand, control and manage their own emotions. Four factors of emotional intelligence have been identified:

1 Well-being
2 Self-control
3 Emotionality
4 Sociability (see Table 8.1).

Resilience

Resilience is associated with the capacity to accurately perceive and respond well to situations that are stressful. Resilience is demonstrated, not only in times of crisis, but on a daily basis.

The Royal College of Nursing suggest that being resilient is about being able to endure setbacks, frustrations and personal misfortunes. During a crisis, the person who is resilient will endeavour to do their best to handle and deal with events calmly, with grace, patience, acceptance and hope. The person who is less resilient may respond with anger, panic, frustration and impatience, and they might see themselves as the victim. Seven key areas that help make a person resilient include the following:

1 Taking care of own basic needs. Making sure you look after yourself and your health and that you are eating well-balanced meals and sleeping well.
2 Having emotional stability. Caring for ill people can bring with it uncomfortable and difficult emotions.
3 Having confidence along with self-esteem, as well as a belief in your ability to manage negative setbacks is at the heart of being resilient.
4 Seeking social support. Strong relationships and support networks are key to coping with challenging situations. People are there to help you and want to help, so ensure you let them.
5 Speaking your truth.
6 Seeking insight. When you come across a challenging situation, regardless of why the situation arose, being aware of what led to it might help you change your behaviour and take a different path next time. Engage with emotional intelligence.
7 Having faith. Difficult situations can often bring a crisis of faith.

As a Nursing Associate, being resilient is important, as caring for people can be physically, mentally, emotionally and spiritually demanding. This can bring with it pressure, and your well-being can suffer.

9 Effective communication

At the point of registration, the Nursing Associate will be able to: communicate effectively using a range of skills and strategies with colleagues and people at all stages of life and with a range of mental, physical, cognitive and behavioural health challenges.

Box 9.1 Communicating with a person who has a cognitive impairment.

When next on a practice placement, take time to consider how someone with a cognitive impairment might find it difficult to understand a care procedure. This could be due to a learning difficulty, dementia, impairment due to a head injury or stroke or a perceptual disturbance due to a psychotic illness.

Identify a particular procedure that you believe may be confusing to the patient, and think of how you can use a variety of different and appropriate communication aids to help the person better understand their care

Box 9.2 Communicating with children and young people and their families.

Observe and take notes (with permission) during a care interaction episode with a child, young person and their family. In particular make notes on how the care interaction episode was terminated: how was it brought to a close?

Consider, for example, how the health or social care professional made verbal and non-verbal signs that the interaction was ending. What was the response of the child, young person and their family? Was an opportunity given for the child, young person and their family to ask questions? Was there any follow-up?

Would you make any changes as to how the interaction was closed, and if so, why? Did you identify any factors that impacted the communication positively?

Communicating with people with chronic and long-term condition

Reflect on one of your practice placements, where a health or social work practitioner had to deliver bad news to a person (and their family) with a chronic and long-term condition. There are several accepted ways to break bad news. Using the mnemonic SPIKES can help. In the grid, did you identify any components of the mnemonic?

Table 9.1 Communication exercise SPIKES (Source: adapted Webb, 2011).

	Your notes
Setting up (Setting the stage for optimal communication)	
Perception (The patient's perception of the news to be shared determines how the news is conveyed).	
Invitation (Permission to have information shared, granted by the patient or family)	
Knowledge (When delivering the news 'Fire a Warning Shot'; let the patient and family know that the incoming news is not good)	
Emotions with Empathy (Emotional response may range from silence to dramatic crying and sobbing; be empathic)	
Strategy or Summary (establish that the patient and family have a clear plan for the future)	

Top Tip

It may sound obvious to say that 'It's how you say it that's important', but this is so true.

The Nursing Associate at a Glance, First Edition. Ian Peate.
© 2021 John Wiley & Sons Ltd. Published 2021 by John Wiley & Sons Ltd.

Effective communication

At the core of everything that is done, everything we do in our work and also outside of work, communication is central. It is key to how we learn, how we perform at work and how we enjoy our non-work interests. Effective communication is especially important when the Nursing Associate and other health and social care professionals offer healthcare and support, where those we offer care and support to (including families) might feel vulnerable, alone, isolated and scared. It is also important because the Nursing Associate works as an integral part of the health and social care team where effective communication is key to helping deliver safe, coordinated and effective care.

Engaging with patients and their families

Every contact counts. All health and social care organisations are responsible for health, well-being, care and safety and each one of us has the opportunity to impact people's mental and physical health and well-being.

At all levels, good, honed communication skills are needed if interventions are to be effective. These interventions begin with the signals that the Nursing Associate gives out when they approach a person; this is even before your interaction has begun. People subconsciously pick up signals from you, and this has the ability to influence whether or not they feel they want to interact with you or not, whether or not they trust you. See Boxes 9.1 and 9.2.

Effective communication

Good communication can help people feel at ease. It is not unusual for people who need health and social care services to express anxieties about their health. They may have anxieties about the variety of tests and investigations they are to undergo, the outcomes of the tests and what the future might hold for them. People react in different ways to stressors or the anxieties that they are facing, and this may sometimes lead them to behave in ways they would not normally behave. For example, they may speak out of character; they might come across as being rude or even aggressive. When the Nursing Associate has effective communication skills and uses them, this can reduce their anxiety, and it can also help to build their confidence.

Connecting with patients

Nursing Associate–patient communication is underpinned by robust interpersonal relationships. When relationships are meaningful, the Nursing Associate can engage the patient in their care. Simple but well-thought-out communication strategies are essential. Table 9.1 provides a range of exercises that may help you become more self-aware and hone the ways in which you care for and approach people.

Making positive connections with patients and others requires the Nursing Associate to listen with attention and to frequently demonstrate to the patient that they have unconditional positive regard for that person.

Unconditional positive regard

By using verbal and non-verbal communication skills, the Nursing Associate can offer the three central requisites of all therapeutic relationships to patients: empathy, genuineness and unconditional positive regard. Having and displaying unconditional positive regards means that you respect the other person as a human being.

Unconditional positive regard involves taking a non-judgemental attitude towards the person, accepting and respecting them for who and what they are. This is not always easy. Unconditional positive regard can be a very difficult skill to learn; it is also, however, a very important one. Sometimes a conflict may arise between the patient's and the Nursing Associate's beliefs and values. It is important to note these differences and conflicts and to develop your helping skills in such a way that any conflict is minimised or, even better, resolved. Any patient in any care setting should be able to feel as if they can freely, without fearing retribution, express their emotions. They should not be made to feel ashamed or humiliated or anxious as to what the Nursing Associate might think of them. The job of the Nursing Associate is to put aside their personal prejudices and offer people a safe and accepting environment.

The Nursing Associate has to put aside any pre-judgements and opinions, accepting the patient at face value and not to allow any judgements that impact the relationship with the patient as this could adversely affect the care and treatment given.

10 Maintaining appropriate relationships

At the point of registration, the Nursing Associate will be able to: demonstrate the skills and abilities required to develop, manage and maintain appropriate relationships with people, their families, carers and colleagues

Figure 10.1   Getting the balance right.

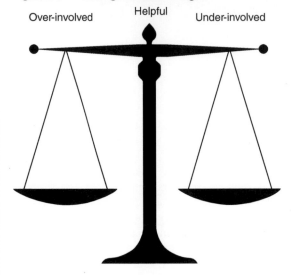

Over-involved   Helpful   Under-involved

Box 10.1   Being helpful and avoiding boundary violation.

Being helpful when implementing care:
- You must treat all patients, at all times with dignity and respect.
- Inspire confidence in patients by speaking, acting and dressing professionally.
- Talk about and treat patients and their families respectfully.
- Be fair and consistent with each patient to inspire trust, amplify your professionalism and enhance your credibility.

Behaviours that should be avoided when planning and implementing patient can include:
- Discussing your intimate or personal issues with a patient
- Keeping secrets with a patient or for a patient
- Spending more time with a patient or re-visiting the patient when you are off-duty or out of uniform
- Engaging in any behaviour that could be misinterpreted as flirting (the Nursing Associate needs to understand the difference between a sincere compliment that has the potential to develop the patient's self-esteem and one that could be understood as flirtatious)
- Taking a patient's side when there is a disagreement between the patient and their spouse or the patient and members of their family.

Box 10.2   The Six Ps and social media.

- Professional – Act professionally at all times.
- Positive – Keep posts positive.
- Person free, patient free – Keep posts person or patient free.
- Protect yourself – Protect your professionalism, your reputation and yourself.
- Privacy – Keep personal and professional lives separate. Check privacy settings and respect privacy of others.
- Pause before you post – Consider the implications of what you are posting. Avoid posting in haste or in anger. Do not respond to other posts in haste.

Top Tip

By virtue of our profession, there are situations in which our designated boundaries permit for intimate entry into another person's/people's life experiences.

The Nursing Associate at a Glance, First Edition. Ian Peate.
© 2021 John Wiley & Sons Ltd. Published 2021 by John Wiley & Sons Ltd.

The Nursing Associate–patient relationship

A therapeutic Nursing Associate–patient relationship is seen as a helping relationship that is based on shared trust and respect. This special caring relationship can develop when the Nursing Associate and the patient come together, and that coming together results in harmony and healing.

Professional boundaries

Professional boundaries define the relationship that supports a therapeutic connection between the Nursing Associate and the patient. Professional boundaries that are encountered in nursing describe a different and more complex kind of relationship than those professional relationships experienced by people in other careers. The professional relationships Nursing Associates share with patients are privileged relationships, and there is a balance that has to be reached between being helpful, under-involved and over-involved (see Figure 10.1).

Because of the profession in which we work, there are a number of situations, encountered day in and day out, in which our designated boundaries allow for intimate entry into another person's life experiences. These professional boundaries are important as they provide guidelines that are essential to us as we practise in a professional manner.

As a result of the knowledge and skills that you possess as a Nursing Associate as well as the privilege you have been afforded in being able to, for example, access confidential information, this makes the patient vulnerable, it gives you power as it is you who controls the care that is provided, you have access to an amazing amount of private and personal information; as well as this, you have specialised nursing knowledge.

Boundary violations

Boundary violations occur when potentially harmful actions breach the Nursing Associate's professional relationship with patients (see Box 10.1). The crossing of boundaries can be blurry, they may not be white or black, they are often grey areas and they may require you to make a professional judgement and indeed to seek the professional advice of others. There are a number of potential violations, including any sexual involvement with a patient.

The crossing of a boundary can have ramifications. A boundary crossing has the potential to damage your relationship with your patient, it can cause harm to other patients, it can put colleagues in difficult and unacceptable situations and also cause risk to your employer and the profession. When boundaries are violated, there is a real risk of legal consequences, and the Nursing and Midwifery Council (NMC) may call you to account for your actions. You may also experience harm as the consequence of your actions could lead to distress, and you might experience negative mental health issues.

When the Nursing Associate carries out their role in a professional manner, they recognise and maintain boundaries so as to establish appropriate limits to relationships. Each Nursing Associate has a responsibility to understand professional boundary guidelines and be aware of the possibility and consequences of violating these boundaries.

Use of social media

The NMC (2019) has produced guidance that sets out broad principles to enable registrants to think through issues and act professionally and ensure public protection at all times. Guidance should be read in conjunction with The Code: Professional Standards of Practice and Behaviour for Nurses, Midwives and Nursing Associates.

When social media is used responsibly and in an appropriate manner, social networking sites can offer several benefits to Nursing Associates. They can use social media to connect with an enormous range of professional development resources as well as locating up-to-date information regarding nursing issues.

The Nursing and Midwifery Board of Ireland discuss six Ps and social media (see Box 10.2).

11 Advocacy and person-centred sensitive care

At the point of registration, the Nursing Associate will be able to: provide, promote and where appropriate advocate for non-discriminatory, person-centred and sensitive care at all times. Reflect on people's values and beliefs, diverse backgrounds, cultural characteristics, language requirements, needs and preferences, taking account any need for adjustments.

Figure 11.1 Eight principles associated with quality improvement (Picker Institute Europe, 2020).

Fast access to reliable health advice

Effective treatment delivered by trusted professionals

Continuity of care and smooth transitions

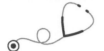

Involvement and support for family and carers

Clear information, communication, and support for self-care

Involvement in decisions and respect for preferences

Emotional support empathy and respect

Attention to physica and environmenta needs

Table 11.1 The four principles of person-centred care (Health Foundation, 2016).

1. Affording people dignity, compassion and respect.
2. Offering coordinated care, support or treatment.
3. Offering personalised care, support or treatment.
4. Supporting people to recognise and develop their own strengths and abilities to enable them to live an independent and fulfilling life.

Table 11.2 PANEL principles (Scottish Human Rights Commission, 2020).

Participation	Everyone has the right to participate in decisions that affect their human rights
Accountability	Effective monitoring as well as effective remedies for breaches in human rights
Non-discrimination and equality	All forms of discrimination must be prohibited, prevented or eliminated
Empowerment	Individuals and communities should know their rights
Legality	Needs to be recognised that rights are legally enforceable

Top Tip

Discrimination is not only offensive – it is also illegal.

The Nursing Associate at a Glance, First Edition. Ian Peate.
© 2021 John Wiley & Sons Ltd. Published 2021 by John Wiley & Sons Ltd.

Person-centred sensitive care

One of the central components of quality healthcare is patient experience. Positive associations have been identified between patient experience, patient safety, clinical effectiveness and a non-discriminatory approach. People's experiences of care provision have to be understood and responded to so as to improve care delivery and quality. The Picker Institute Europe (2019) have identified eight Principles of Person-Centred Care that provide a quality improvement framework. These principles can be used to enable individuals and organisations to understand the experiences of those who use services and staff so as to assist with quality improvement (see Figure 11.1).

Towards a Definition

There is no single agreed definition of the term 'person-centred care'. This concept is used to refer to several different principles and activities. Person-centred care is very much a dynamic, fluid concept. If the Nursing Associate is to offer care that is person centred, then what this looks like will very much depend on individual needs, unique circumstances and the personal preferences of the person receiving care. What might be important to one person with regards to their health and well-being needs may be unnecessary, or even unacceptable, to another. It should also be remembered that individual needs may change over time. The Health Foundation (2016) has identified a framework that embraces four Principles of Person-Centred Care (see Table 11.1).

Whenever the Nursing Associate is offering care to people, this should be guided by the principles outlined in Figure 11.1 and Table 11.1. The provision of person-centred care, within any healthcare experience, involves a combination of these guiding principles, along with adherence to the tenets outlined in the Code.

Advocacy

The roles of the Nursing Associate are varied and complex, and acting as an advocate is one of those roles. Underpinning all chapters of this text is the therapeutic Nursing Associate–patient relationship. This relationship, a helping relationship that is steeped in trust, is a special relationship that should never be taken for granted. The Nursing Associate at all times is required to provide, promote and where appropriate advocate for non-discriminatory, person-centred and sensitive care. This has to take into account people's values and beliefs, their backgrounds, cultural characteristics, language requirements, their needs and preferences and to make any adjustments where necessary.

In order to provide contemporary care, there is a need for fundamental changes in how health and social care professionals deliver care. An important change requires ensuring the delivery of care, treatment offered and services provided reflects a rights-based approach, which requires that the person is at the centre of all we do. In advocating for people, the challenge is to positively manage risk and deliver care amid complex legal and ethical processes that have to guide practice.

A rights-based approach means advocating for those who are in need and providing people with greater opportunities to participate in shaping the decisions that impact them (their human rights). It also means increasing the ability of those with responsibility for fulfilling rights to recognise and know how to respect those rights and make sure they can be held to account. The PANEL principles (Table 11.2) highlight some underlying principles which are of fundamental importance in applying a human-rights-based approach in practice.

In all of its guises, advocacy should aim to ensure that people, particularly those in our society who are most vulnerable, are able to have their voice heard on issues that they consider important to them, defend and safeguard their rights and have their views and their wishes genuinely considered when decisions are being made about their lives. For those people who cannot articulate their views about their care and treatment, regardless of the reason, advocacy is an important approach by which a person can be considered and protected in what can be very complex decision-making about how they wish to live their lives and how their care is provided.

A relative or carer can be an advocate; someone close to the person, representing what the person would decide if they were able to make their own decisions. A Nursing Associate or health and social care professional could be an advocate for a person who has no one else, supporting them in understanding what is being proposed about their care and treatment. Advocacy services are also available. An external organisation can provide a person with expertise in representing the views of those who cannot do so independently, helping in decision-making processes.

Reporting adverse incidents

At the point of registration, the Nursing Associate will be able to: recognise and report any factors that may adversely impact safe and effective care provision.

Box 12.1 Being open and honest when something goes wrong with treatment or care.

- Inform the patient (or, where appropriate, the patient's advocate, carer or family) when something has gone wrong.
- Apologise to the patient (or, where appropriate, the patient's advocate, carer or family).
- Offer an appropriate remedy or support to put matters right (if possible).
- Explain fully to the patient (or, where appropriate, the patient's advocate, carer or family) the short- and long-term effects of what has happened.

Table 12.1 Encouraging the reporting of adverse incidents.

Encourage reporting	Report even minor incidents and 'near misses'; this is just as important as major events in identifying and analysing problems with safety.
Analyse all factors involved, not just the actions of one individual	Incidents rarely have one cause; most are almost always multifactorial. All institutional issues should be included in the analysis.
Analyse results logically, formulate action plans	Identify the cause of the incident. Focus on the story and all the contributory issues, not on the individual. Look for all the underlying causes, not just the 'final error' leading to the incident. Devise action plans addressing the issues.
Feed back the results of the process	Those reporting incidents should be informed of the results of the investigation and actions taken. Key action points should be shared with all staff members
Take action to prevent future incidents	It will take time for staff to accept that reporting incidents will not land them in trouble. When they see visible changes and staff are made aware that their commitment to safety is valued, most staff will embrace the reporting system.
Promote a team approach	Make clear that everyone has a key role to play. Ensure staff feel valued, and support those experiencing stress due to being involved in a clinical incident.

Top Tip

Patient safety is everyone's business. Adverse events can be prevented through screening and early identification of the factors that put people at risk.

The Nursing Associate at a Glance, First Edition. Ian Peate.
© 2021 John Wiley & Sons Ltd. Published 2021 by John Wiley & Sons Ltd.

Safety and effective care

It is everyone's responsibility to ensure safety in healthcare. The Code requires all Nursing Associates to promote patient safety. Day in and day out in our NHS, tens of thousands of patients are treated safely by staff who are dedicated and motivated to provide high-quality and safe clinical care. For most patients, the treatment received alleviates or improves symptoms, and their experience is a positive one.

Despite this, critical incidents that destroy people's lives are a reality, and patient safety is still an ongoing and critical challenge.

Safety and effectiveness is a fundamental principle of delivering care, regardless of the setting or the types of people who are using the service.

Safe care occurs when people who use and deliver health or social care services are free from unnecessary or potential harm associated with the delivery of the services. Harm may be physical, psychological and/or emotional. When a person's care and treatment is said to be effective, it is appropriate for their needs, delivered by the right person who has the right skills and experience, delivered in the right place and at the right time. It is more than doing no harm; it is about doing something that achieves a positive outcome and experience for the person and, if appropriate, their families too.

Adverse incidents

An adverse incident (also known as an adverse event) is an incident resulting in harm to the patient. Adverse events are commonly experienced by patients over 70 years and include falls, medication errors, malnutrition, incontinence and hospital-acquired pressure injuries and infections.

What the Nursing Associate does or does not do to identify and respond to issues such as malnutrition, uncontrolled pain and unrecognised delirium can contribute to a patient experiencing an adverse event and in turn functional decline.

Contemporary treatment options are powerful and complex; those who provide healthcare face many pressures with regard to their workloads, adverse events or incidents occur across health and social care settings.

Human error and unsafe procedures and equipment often underlie many of the incidents which occur. Everyone makes mistakes; however, critical incidents are rarely caused by one person alone. Often, they are due to a combination of factors.

All too often the same errors have been made repeatedly. This means that healthcare staff tend not to report mistakes or 'near misses' (errors or disasters narrowly avoided), fearing that if they do they may be blamed and punished.

Whilst it may be impossible to prevent errors, it is, however, possible, to put in place procedures that can act as barriers to making mistakes. It is important to raise concerns so that problems occurring can be identified and precautions can be taken against recurrence. If, for example, there are no reports of medication errors, then no one will know that manufacturing, dispensing and prescribing errors are occurring (and they do occur).

It is essential, therefore, to implement a completely open system of reporting of all adverse incidents and near misses (see Table 12.1).

Reporting

Health and social care organisations have policies for reporting adverse incidents and near misses, and the Nursing Associate is required to follow these. Various reporting systems and schemes are used for reporting adverse incidents and near misses. The Nursing Associate must also comply with any system in the organisation for reporting adverse incidents that put patient safety at risk. Do not try to prevent colleagues or former colleagues from raising concerns about patient safety.

Duty of Candour

Candour is defined by the Care Council of Wales as the volunteering of all relevant information to persons who have, or may have, been harmed by the provision of services, whether or not the information has been requested and whether or not a complaint or a report about that provision has been made. See also Chapter 3.

If a mistake has been made, be open and honest about it (Box 12.1). This includes providing a full and prompt explanation to your manager or employer of what has happened.

The Nursing Associate should apologise to the individual for what happened. An apology is not an admission of legal liability, but the individual has the right to receive an apology from the most appropriate team member. Record the details of the apology in the individual's records.

13 Numeracy, literacy, digital and technological skills

At the point of registration, the Nursing Associate will be able to: demonstrate the numeracy, literacy, digital and technological skills required to meet the needs of people in their care to ensure safe and effective practice.

Figure 13.1 Digital literacies.

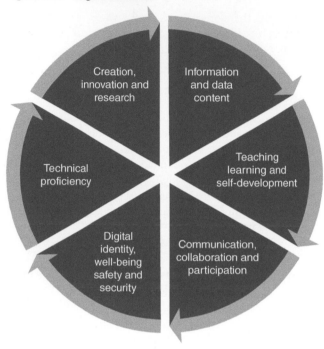

Creation, innovation and research

Information and data content

Technical proficiency

Teaching learning and self-development

Digital identity, well-being safety and security

Communication, collaboration and participation

Box 13.1 Suggestions to enhance confidence in relation to numeracy and maths.

- Practice – Maths. As is the case with other skills, the less it is used the more likely it is to be forgotten.
- Practice is the most direct way of improving skills and fostering confidence. Take your time. Do not feel rushed when handling a number of problems at work.
- Take time – Take the time you need to be confident in your answers, and ask for help if you need help. Ask a colleague to check calculations at work, or seek support outside of work to improve your skills.
- There is a wide range of freely available online maths resources.

Table 13.1 The PEACE mnemonic.

Plan	What are you trying to do? Before you begin, consider the type of problem you are trying to solve. What are you looking for?
Estimate	What does a sensible answer look like? Prior to calculating it is important to think about (estimate) what a sensible answer might be.
Approach	How are you going to solve the problem? What method of calculation are you going to use? What steps are involved in the calculation?
Calculate	When undertaking a calculation, consider these important points: • Check each step • Do not rush • Take your time • Do not feel pressured • When using a calculator, take care.
Evaluate	Do not skip this step. After making the calculation, it needs to be checked. Ask yourself: 'Does this answer look right? Does it fit the estimated answer I came up with in my estimation?' If concerned, check again

When using a calculator, remember that it only responds to the numbers you put in it; if a mistake is made entering numbers, the answer you get will be wrong.

Top Tip

It is important to note that the only way to ensure that patients receive the correct amount of medications is to perform the calculation correctly or to seek help and advice if you are unsure how to do this. The calculation of a drug dose must never be guessed.

The Nursing Associate at a Glance, First Edition. Ian Peate.
© 2021 John Wiley & Sons Ltd. Published 2021 by John Wiley & Sons Ltd.

A key feature of the Nursing Associate's role is to be able to demonstrate proficiency with regard to numeracy, literacy and digital and technological skills so as to undertake a range of functions. These activities take place daily in health and social care settings.

Numeracy

Numeracy is important in health and social care, playing a vital role in a variety of arenas. The safe administration of medicines is but one area.

The Nursing Associate is required to discuss medical conditions with colleagues and patients, and as they do this they are interpreting information, writing formal and informal reports, identifying patterns and trends in numbers (for example, a change in a patient's condition), reading numerical information from medical equipment (e.g. pulse oximeters, blood pressure), administering medicines, taking measurements and accurately recording results (e.g. blood results).

In order to do all of this in a safe and effective way, the Nursing Associate will need to improve and develop mathematical skills so as to enhance care provision and confidence. The Nursing Associate is required to possess the necessary numerical competence to deliver care to the standard required.

Maths is a skill that anyone can improve with practice. Box 13.1 provides suggestions for ways in which the Nursing Associate can develop skills, reduce anxiety and enhance confidence in this area. The PEACE mnemonic can be used to help you succeed when faced with numeracy challenges (see Table 13.1).

It is useful to ask a colleague to double-check a calculation if you have even the slightest worry about your result. Anyone can make a simple error on a particular day. There may be a policy in your workplace that every calculation must always be double-checked when dispensing medicines.

Literacy

It is essential that the Nursing Associate and other health and social care professionals ensure that they keep good written records regarding care provided. There are a variety of reasons for this, for example, to ensure care and treatment can continue to be given safely regardless of which staff are on duty, 24 hours a day, seven days a week; to record the care given to the patient and to make sure there is an accurate record that may be used at a later date, for example, if there is a complaint about care received.

Digital and technological skills

Information and technology is transforming the way health and care services are being designed and delivered. The opportunities are significant, and the innovation and commitment to change in many areas is making a real difference to people's lives.

Information and technology have the potential to support people in hospitals and also to allow them to live at home longer, enabling professionals to work effectively together across multiple organisations. The Nursing Associate must develop and update the skills needed to ensure full use of information and technology, for the benefit of the patient.

There are many examples of transformation enabled by information and technology. Technology will not be a replacement for care; it can, however, support individuals receiving health and social care, carers or professionals delivering care.

Information and technology plays a key part in the delivery of care. If we are to maximise the benefits that it can bring and utilise it to the maximum, engagement and collaboration will be required from across systems locally and nationally. In particular, the statutory, voluntary and community sectors have to work together with a shared purpose.

Digital literacies

Becoming and developing further as a digitally literate Nursing Associate will involve expanding on the skills, attitudes, values and behaviours detailed in Figure 13.1.

Digital identity, well-being and safety: Managing personal and professional identities.

Information, data and media literacies: Support others to find reliable information, use technology to coordinate care. Appreciating how data is structured within health record systems, conform to legal, professional requirements.

Teaching, learning and self-development: Participate in learning, and use digital media/tools.

Communication, collaboration and participation: Use appropriate forms of communication, respect points of view and cultural differences.

Technical proficiency: Competently use devices, applications and software.

Digital creation, innovation and scholarship: Work with others to co-design and co-develop digitally enabled ways of working, shaping the research agenda.

14 Record keeping

At the point of registration, the Nursing Associate will be able to: demonstrate the ability to keep complete, clear, accurate and timely records.

Box 14.1 Retention of records.

In England the Records Management Code https://tinyurl.com/y5vyouc2 outlines the retention periods for people working with or in the NHS. In summary, they are as follows:

- GP Records – 10 years after death or after leaving the UK (unless they remain in the EU). Electronic patient records must be stored for the foreseeable future.
- Maternity Records – 25 years after the birth of the last child.
- Children and Young People – until the patient's 25th birthday or 8 years after their death.
- Mental Health Records – 20 years or 8 years after their death.

Box 14.2 Good record keeping.

- Handwrite legibly and key in competently to computer systems.
- Sign all entries.
- Record events accurately and clearly. The patient may wish to see the record at some point, so write in a language that the patient will understand.
- Focus on facts; do not speculate.
- Avoid unnecessary abbreviations.
- Record how the patient is contributing to their care. Quote anything they have said that you think may be significant.
- Never change or alter anything someone else has written, or change anything you have written previously; if you need to amend something you have written, draw a clear line through it, and sign and date the changes.
- Never write anything about a patient or colleague that is insulting or derogatory.

Table 14.1 Using the four senses.

Sight	Feel
Mannerism, body movements, bleeding, the colour of urine, what is seen in vomitus, pallor, sweating, bruises, oedema, sores/lesions, redness, the colour of body fluid, pupil reaction, use of space, rash	Crepitus, rigidity, muscle strength, moisture, localised heat/cold, pulse, palpation, oedema
Smell	**Hear**
Faecal odours, urine odours, fruity odours, foul-smelling drainage, some microorganisms' infections have specific identifiable odours, alcohol breath	Crying, breathing, wheezing, heart and lung sounds, bowel sounds

Top Tip

When caring for a patient, it is important to ensure good record keeping to promote patient care and improve communication. Good record keeping is the result of effective teamwork and is an important tool that helps to develop high-quality healthcare and reinforces professionalism within nursing.

The Nursing Associate at a Glance, First Edition. Ian Peate.
© 2021 John Wiley & Sons Ltd. Published 2021 by John Wiley & Sons Ltd.

The Nursing and Midwifery Council (NMC) require all Nursing Associates to communicate effectively, and one element of this is to keep clear and accurate records which are relevant to their practice. Good record keeping is a fundamental aspect of nursing. A care record is seen as any paper or electronic-based record containing information or personal data concerning people's care.

Keeping clear and accurate records

Maintaining clear and accurate records applies to the records relevant to your scope of practice. This includes but is not limited to patient records. In order to achieve this requirement, the Nursing Associate must complete records at the time, or if this is not possible, as soon as possible after an event, recording if the notes are written sometime after the event occurred. Identify risks or problems that have occurred and steps taken to deal with them, so that colleagues who use the records will have all the information they require. Records must be completed accurately, without any falsification, taking immediate and appropriate action if you become aware that someone has not adhered to these requirements. Ensure that you attribute any entries you make in paper or electronic records to yourself. Be sure they are written clearly, dated and timed. Do not include any unnecessary abbreviations, jargon or speculation. All records must be kept securely. You must collect, treat and store all data (including digital data) and research findings appropriately. At all times adhere to local policy and procedure. The Nursing Associate must ensure they are clear concerning their responsibilities for record keeping, regardless of the format in which they are kept. There is a system to dispose of care records appropriately; they may also need to be destroyed (see Box 14.1).

Countersigning records

Record keeping can be delegated to a number of health and social care providers including health care assistants, assistant practitioners, trainee Nursing Associates, nursing apprentices and nursing students so that they are able to document the care provided.

However, as this is a delegated activity, as with any other delegated activity, the person delegating the activity (for example, the Nursing Associate) must ensure that the person being delegated to (for example, a trainee Nursing Associate) is competent to undertake the activity and that it is in the patient's best interests for record keeping to be delegated. Supervision and a countersignature will be required until the person being delegated to is competent at keeping records. The Nursing Associate should only countersign if they have observed the activity or can confirm it had taken place.

Good record keeping

Anything you write by hand or enter using electronic systems must be honest, accurate and non-offensive; you must not breach patient confidentiality. When these four principles are followed, any contribution that is made to record keeping will be valuable. Handwritten records should be written in black ink, so that if required they can be photocopied. Good record-keeping points are made in Box 14.2.

Being objective is an important feature of good record keeping. State facts from what you have seen, felt, heard and smelt. Recording sensory observations helps to discriminate between fact (objectivity) – which is what has truly happened – and opinion (subjectivity) – which is what could have, may have happened. Table 14.1 considers the four senses.

An important feature of the record-keeping process is the storage of records. Records must be returned to locked storage as soon as possible; they should not be left in an office, in a car or in individual homes. Do not leave computer records on screens as they could be viewed by unauthorised staff or members of the public.

Legal standards

At any point, records, documents and photographs related to care provision could be taken by the police or by the coroner. They may be requested by the patient and/or the patient's family for use in litigation and therefore by the courts, or by regulators or inspectors during an examination of care provided, all of whom will scrutinise the evidence within those records, documents and photographs.

The Nursing Associate may be called to account for their previous practice, often several years later, and previous documentation may be required for this purpose. It is therefore not only in the patient's interests but also in the care provider's interests to maintain high standards of documentation at all times. The Nursing Associate may be required to produce documentary evidence of the care provided to every patient they are responsible for.

15 Reflective practice

At the point of registration, the Nursing Associate will be able to: take responsibility for continuous self-reflection, seeking and responding to support and feedback to develop professional knowledge and skills.

Table 15.1 Three components associated with reflection.

1. Reflection before action	Requires the Nursing Associated to think about what you aim to achieve and understanding how this will be achieved by using previous experience.
2. Reflection in action	Considers your conduct while carrying out the task, permitting you to modify what you are doing as you are doing it. Often described as 'thinking on your feet'.
3. Reflection on action	Involves retrospective analysis of how practice was carried out and analysing the information gathered with respect to knowledge, new learning and professional development.

Figure 15.1   A reflective process.

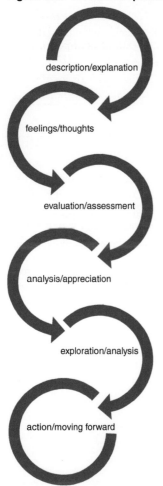

description/explanation

feelings/thoughts

evaluation/assessment

analysis/appreciation

exploration/analysis

action/moving forward

Top Tip
Reflective practice is a form of ongoing learning as the Nursing Associate examines what happens in their setting and reflects on what they could change or develop.

The Nursing Associate at a Glance, First Edition. Ian Peate.

Reflective practice

Effective reflective practice requires the Nursing Associate to make sense of events, situations and actions that happen in the workplace. Refection is a process and should be undertaken using a structure.

The process of reflection invites the Nursing Associate to look back at significant events that have occurred in the workplace (see Figure 15.1); it encourages you to:

- Explain what happened, what the event was about (description/explanation)
- Consider how the event made you feel (feelings/thoughts)
- Undertake an assessment of what was good and what was bad about the event (evaluation/assessment)
- Take stock of the event so you can get an overall appreciation of its importance (analysis/appreciation)
- Think about how things might have been done in a different way (exploration/analysis)
- Consider how you might act if a similar event presented itself in the future (action/moving forward).

Reflective writing offers an opportunity to gain further insight from the work you do through deeper reflection on experiences and through further consideration of other perspectives from people and theory. When we undertake reflective practice, we can deepen the learning from the work we do.

When adopting this approach to reflection, one needs to critically review experience from practice so that it can be used to inform and change future practice in a positive way. In examining practice, the Nursing Associate needs to be authentic, openly examining how they are practising, to be courageous, open-minded and to develop a willingness to accept and act on feedback.

Definitions

A number of authors (for example, Schön 1983; Rolfe et al. 2010) have attempted to define reflection. As reflection is a very personal activity, there are several definitions. It seems, however, that there are three components associated with reflection (see Table 15.1):

1 Reflection before action
2 Reflection in action
3 Reflection on action.

Models of reflection

There are many models of reflection that can be used in and for nursing practice/education. Whilst the structure and format of the models differ, the underlying principles will be the same. A model offers a systematic and structured approach. Applying a reflective model can help you focus on learning and self-awareness after an event has occurred. It helps you avoid simply retelling the events, telling a story. The model you choose is usually based on personal preference.

The Nursing and Midwifery Council (NMC) and reflection

Reflective practice and reflection are lifelong skills that can be honed, developed and adapted to a number of situations and can meet a range of requirements.

The NMC state that reflection is a key element of development and educational requirements and it is also a condition for revalidation; the principles of reflection apply to everyone on the register. Nursing Associates are encouraged to engage in reflective practice and to foster a culture of sharing, reflection and improvement' this can help to prevent the Nursing Associate from practising in professional isolation.

When revalidating, the Nursing Associate must provide five written reflective accounts and a reflective discussion with another nurse, midwife or Nursing Associate on the register.

The reflective accounts have to be based on either instances of (or a combination of) continuous professional development, feedback or an event or experience that has occurred in practice. The discussion should be from the three-year period since the Nursing Associate last renewed or joined the register. Discussion should reflect on positive and constructive experiences, explaining what was learnt, how practice has changed or how practice has improved as a result and how this all links to the four key themes of the Code.

16 Promoting public confidence in the profession

At the point of registration, the Nursing Associate will be able to: act as an ambassador for their profession and promote public confidence in health and care services.

Figure 16.1 The Code.

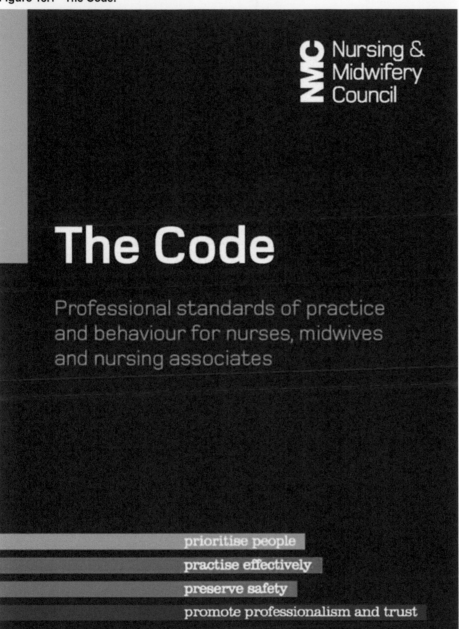

NMC Nursing & Midwifery Council

The Code

Professional standards of practice and behaviour for nurses, midwives and nursing associates

prioritise people

practise effectively

preserve safety

promote professionalism and trust

Top Tip
Good health and care outcomes are very much related to the professional practice and behaviours of Nursing Associates.

Professionalism

Professionalism means something to everyone who works as a Nursing Associate. It means being an inspiring role model working in the best interests of people you offer care to, regardless of the position held or where you practise.

The ultimate purpose of professionalism in nursing is to ensure the provision of consistent safe, effective, person-centred outcomes that will support people and their families and carers, so as to achieve an optimal status of health and well-being.

The Code

The Code: Professional Standards of Practice and Behaviour for Nurses, Midwives and Nursing Associates published by the Nursing and Midwifery Council (2018; see Figure 16.1) represents the professional standards that all Nursing Associates are required to uphold if they wish to be registered and to practise in the UK. The Code is arranged around four themes:

1 Prioritise people
2 Practise effectively
3 Preserve safety
4 Promote professionalism and trust.

See also Chapter 1.

The Code was created by people who care about good-quality nursing and midwifery. The Nursing Associate can use the Code as a way of reinforcing and demonstrating their professionalism. If the Nursing Associate fails to adhere to the tenets within the Code, their fitness to practise may be brought into question.

Whether a patient is having an operation or having investigations at their general practice or local clinic, they want to receive good nursing care, feel safe, looked after and listened to, they will also want the same to apply to their relatives. It makes no difference if the delivery of care occurs at a GP surgery, hospital, place of detention, care home or in the person's own home.

Good care

When providing good care, acting as an ambassador for the profession and promoting public confidence in health and care, the Nursing Associate:

- Must be kind and respectful, putting care and safety first, encouraging the patient to take part in decisions about their care.
- Listens to patients and pays attention to any concerns, respecting the person's right to dignity, privacy and confidentiality.
- Is open and honest about care and any treatment provided, ensuring the patient is safe, reducing, as far they possible, the risk of any mistakes and harm. If mistakes do happen, the Nursing Associate offers an apology, explaining what has happened as well as the likely effects.
- Demonstrates, at all times, honesty and integrity, raising any concerns straightaway if there is any belief that the patient is vulnerable, at risk or in need of extra support and protection. Action will be taken if there are any concerns about the care and safety of patients.
- Pays attention to the patient's well-being, as well as treatment and care, helping the patient to access the care and support that they require.

The Royal College of Nursing (2013) have developed eight principles/statements that describe what constitutes safe and effective nursing care. These apply to all nursing staff, regardless of the care setting, for example, Nursing Associates, ward managers in hospitals, team leaders in community, specialist nurses, community nurses, health visitors, healthcare assistants, Trainee Nursing Associates and student nurses. The principles address aspects of behaviour, attitude and approach that all underpin professional practice. The Nursing Associate:

- Treats everyone in their care with dignity and humanity.
- Takes responsibility for the care they provide and answers for their own judgements and actions.
- Manages risk, is vigilant about risk, keeping everyone safe in the places they receive health care.
- Provides and promotes care that puts people at the centre of all that is done.
- Is at the heart of the communication process.
- Has up-to-date knowledge and skills.
- Works closely with their own team and with other professionals, making sure patients' care and treatment is coordinated.
- Leads by example, develops themselves and others.

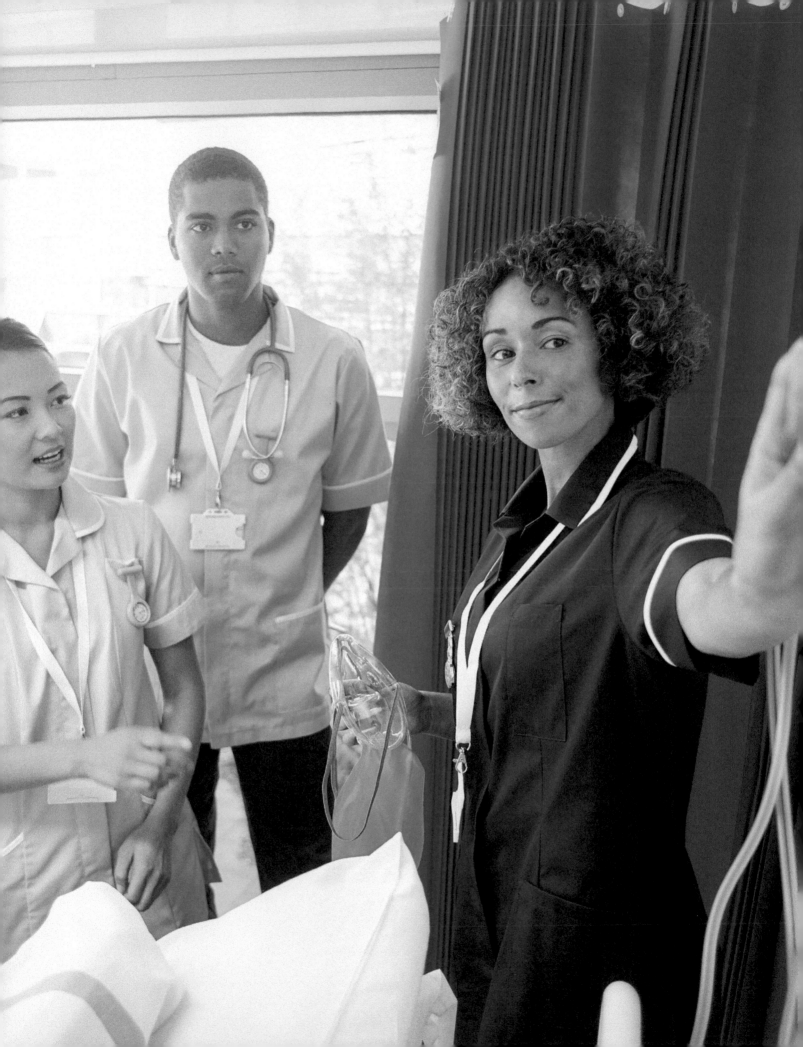

Promoting health and preventing ill health

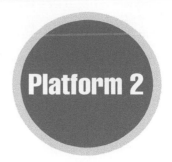

Platform 2

Chapters

17 Principles of health promotion

At the point of registration, the Nursing Associate will be able to: understand and apply the aims and principles of health promotion, protection and improvement and the prevention of ill health when engaging with people.

Figure 17.1   The Stages of Change Model.

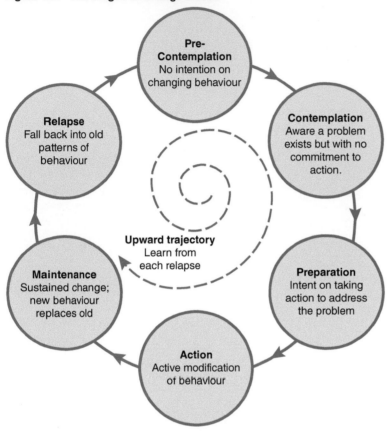

Top Tip

The factors which influence health are multiple and interactive. They are the determinants of health. They are a range of personal, social, economic and environmental factors determining the health status of individuals or populations.

The Nursing Associate at a Glance, First Edition. Ian Peate.
© 2021 John Wiley & Sons Ltd. Published 2021 by John Wiley & Sons Ltd.

Health promotion and health education

Health promotion provides opportunities for individuals, communities and populations to understand the determinants (these are the influences) of their health and well-being and how they can be improved.

Health promotion is different from health education, and often the two are inadvertently used synonymously. Health education tends to focus primarily on the giving of information in order to change health behaviours. Health education is explaining to people the facts of what health is, in clear and identifiable terms, and teaching people exercise to improve their balance and reduce weight and improve their sexual health. It is important that the Nursing Associate considers health education and the focus this takes.

Health promotion is a term that is applied to a range of approaches that are designed to improve the health of people, communities and populations. It involves the empowerment of individuals and aims to alter attitudes that may result in health behaviour changes.

Definition

The WHO Health Promotion Glossary 1998 provides a definition of health promotion: it is the process of enabling people to increase control over and to improve their health. The definition came about after the first International Conference on Health Promotion was held in Ottawa in 1986, launching a number of actions among international organisations, national governments and local communities to achieve the goal of 'Health for All' by the year 2000 and beyond. The key principles of strategies for health promotion identified in the Ottawa Charter were:

- Advocate (to enhance the factors which encourage health)
- Enable (allowing all to achieve health equity)
- Facilitate (through collaboration and partnership) across all sectors.

Health promotion is a public health approach that is based on the notion that there are significant health gains to be made from encouraging people to live healthier, fitter and more active lives, avoiding known risks to health. The interventions used by health promotion are focussed on helping people to make healthier choices for themselves. In health promotion, the focus is on health and not illness. It is also on the involvement of people, groups and communities in helping themselves.

Health promotion models and approaches

Health promotion is not something that the Nursing Associate 'does to' people; it is usually undertaken alongside their other roles and functions. Health promotion can be absorbed into everyday work activity, making every contact with patients and/or relatives count, taking these contacts as an opportunity to look at health issues working in partnership.

There are a number of theories and models that support the practice of health promotion and disease prevention. The models are used to help understand and explain health behaviour and to guide the identification, development and implementation of interventions. When choosing a model to guide health promotion, it is important to consider a number of factors, for example, the specific health problem being addressed, the population(s) that are being served as well as the contexts in which the activity is being implemented.

The Stages of Change model

This is but one model that is available (see Figure 17.1). This model describes the different stages that people go through when they want to change something in their everyday lives.

Pre-contemplation: The person may ask what the problem is. People do not want to admit that they have a problem; they prefer to avoid any consideration of the subject.

Contemplation: The person is beginning to think about their behaviour, becoming aware of problems.

Preparation/determination: The person has realised that something needs to change and are ready to make changes – but they may not know how exactly.

Action: At this stage, the person knows that they want to change, and they take the plunge, beginning to understand how they can change. Aims and targets are set.

Maintenance: Maintaining this stage requires the person to 'stick with it' and sustain their new, healthier lifestyle.

Relapse: This is part of the model, an acknowledgement that the person may revert to their old ways. It includes learning from any relapse.

18 Health behaviours

At the point of registration, the Nursing Associate will be able to: promote preventive health behaviours and provide information to support people to make informed choices to improve their mental, physical, behavioural health and well-being.

Figure 18.1 Factors impacting health behaviours.

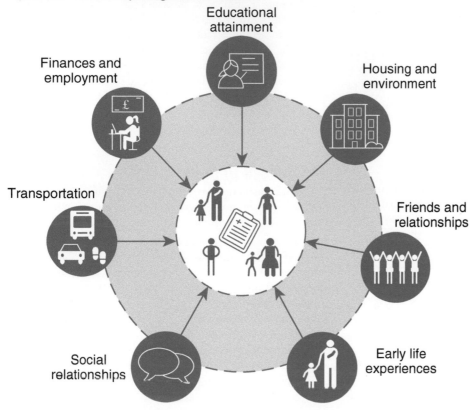

Top Tip
Lifestyle-related diseases such as diabetes, cardiovascular disease and some cancers represent the greatest global health threat.

Definition

In 1997 Gochman defined health behaviours as '. . . overt behavioural patterns, actions and habits that relate to health maintenance, to health restoration and to health improvement'.

There are several behaviours that this definition encompasses, including:

- Smoking
- Alcohol use
- Diet
- Physical activity
- Sexual behaviours
- Adherence to medication
- Screening
- Vaccination.

Health behaviours and the issue of health behaviours should be considered by the Nursing Associate in both healthy and unhealthy populations. This is an important area, and it can and has made worthy contributions to improving health.

It is important to note that health behaviours do not occur in isolation. They are influenced and constrained by a number of social and cultural norms (see Figure 18.1).

Health behaviours

Helping people tackle a range of behaviours such as smoking, alcohol misuse, poor eating patterns and lack of physical activity can have much potential for improving health and well-being. These behaviours are linked to health problems and chronic diseases, for example, cardiovascular disease, type 2 diabetes and cancer. The interventions that are used to help people change can include:

- Improving diet and become more physically active
- Losing weight if the person is overweight or obese
- Stopping smoking
- Reducing alcohol intake
- Practising safer sex.

Health behaviours are influenced by the social, cultural and physical environments in which people live and work, and they are affected by individual choices and external constraints. Positive behaviours can help to promote health and prevent disease; the opposite, however, is true for risk behaviours. When health behaviours are observed over time, it is possible to anticipate risk to population health, identify those sectors of the population who are most in need of public health intervention and to undertake an evaluation of the effectiveness of public health policies and practices.

Patterns of behaviour

There are differences in patterns of health behaviours among, for example, gender, with men being more likely than females to smoke and to drink heavily. They are also less likely to eat enough fruit and vegetables. Sleep disturbance is found in both genders however, more so in females.

Gender

Social roles that are traditionally attributed to women and men are relevant in gender differences with regard to health and well-being. Gender plays a significant role in the patterns of health information behaviour, and the Nursing Associate needs to take this into consideration when designing health promotion materials and offering intervention programmes and activities. More research is needed in this area before these very complex gender-related circumstances can be fully understood.

Age

Differences in behaviour can also be related to age. Younger people (particularly men) are more likely to engage in risky health behaviours, whereas increased age predicts more protective health behaviour. Older people tend to eat more fruit and vegetables and have lower levels of smoking and excessive drinking.

Education

People who have received more formal education are the least likely to smoke, and they are the most likely to be physically active in middle age. They also tend to make healthy changes overall and more consistently adhere to them. Education also shapes behavioural change after a new diagnosis is made, which is likely to contribute to socio-economic status differences in chronic disease management and health outcomes.

19 Epidemiology, demography and genomics

At the point of registration, the Nursing Associate will be able to: describe the principles of epidemiology, demography and genomics and how these may influence health and well-being outcomes.

Table 19.1 Genomics glossary of terms.

Gene	The unit of heredity, a section of genetic sequence encoding one protein
Genome	The entire genetic material of an organism – the blueprint for life
Genomics	Study of the structure, function, evolution, mapping of and editing of genomes

Table 19.2 Genomic versus genetics.

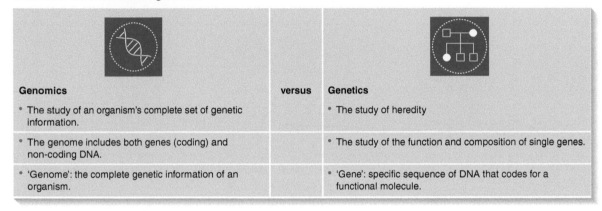

Genomics	versus	Genetics
• The study of an organism's complete set of genetic information.		• The study of heredity
• The genome includes both genes (coding) and non-coding DNA.		• The study of the function and composition of single genes.
• 'Genome': the complete genetic information of an organism.		• 'Gene': specific sequence of DNA that codes for a functional molecule.

Figure 19.1 Demographics.

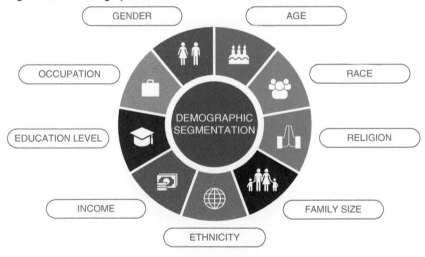

Top Tip

The Nursing Associate is central to the public's health, whether delivering screening programmes, annual health checks or simply the numerous points of contact they have with patients during their lifetime.

The Nursing Associate at a Glance, First Edition. Ian Peate.
© 2021 John Wiley & Sons Ltd. Published 2021 by John Wiley & Sons Ltd.

Providing care to people in a way that is meaningful and has impact requires the Nursing Associate to understand patterns in healthcare and the progression of diseases, and the conditions that produce good health and social care as well as those that hinder it. Clinical practice is influenced by epidemiology, demography and genomics.

Epidemiology

Epidemiology is the science of counting health events in public health, allowing us to understand those conditions that produce health and social care issues and the distribution of health within and across populations. It is the study of how often diseases occur in various populations of people and why, and it helps us to understand those factors that promote good health and how good health is distributed. It also has the potential to help us appreciate those dynamics that can result in poor health. Epidemiology is at the heart of public health.

The data that epidemiologists produce make it possible for us to analyse further the determinants of health. Epidemiology is uniquely quantitative, providing hard data and opportunities to quantify the drivers of health and states of health locally, nationally and globally.

Two of the key concepts of epidemiology are prevalence and incidence. Prevalence looks at existing cases, i.e. cases already existing in the population, and is usually expressed as a fraction (for example, 1/3), as a percentage (%) or as the number of cases per 10,000 or 100,000 people. Prevalence can be measured at a particular point in time (point prevalence), or over a specified period such as a year (period prevalence).

Incidence is the number of new cases of a health event (such as development of a disease, or reaction to a medicine) occurring during a specific time period, usually a year, in a specified population. Incidence therefore is also a measure of the risk of experiencing the health event during a certain period of time. See Figure 19.1.

Demography

Demographics are defined as statistical data about the characteristics of a population, for example, the age, gender and income of the people within the population (see Figure 19.1). Information is also available on the lifestyle, employment status, accident rate and density of population per region.

The process of studying the local population is extremely important. It can enable data to be gathered, offering information about specific populations. Once that data is available, it can illustrate the changing structures of populations, allowing targeted responses to be made to health and social care needs in a more meaningful way.

When the Nursing Associate is aware of the configuration of a local population, they will have a much better chance of engaging with those people and delivering public health initiatives. For example, if the data reveals high levels of smokers or people with alcohol abuse issues in the area, the Nursing Associate could tailor a stop smoking or alcohol awareness campaign and know that the local population would identify with this.

Genomics

It is defined as the branch of molecular biology that is concerned with the structure, function, evolution and mapping of genomes (see Table 19.1).

Genomic information is important for a number of areas in public health protection, from the tracking of infectious disease outbreaks, to identifying inherited disorders and characterising mutations that underpin the progression of cancers.

Like genetics, genomics also looks at DNA. The key difference between genomics and genetics is that genetics scrutinises the functioning and composition of the single gene; genomics however, addresses all genes and their inter-relationships so as to identify their combined influence on the growth and development of the organism (see Table 19.2). This is leading to changes in the way we diagnose, treat and care for patients and their families. There are many applications for genomics in nursing.

As the understanding of genomics develops, this can lead to better diagnosis, management and the potential to even prevent a range of health conditions, bringing long-awaited answers where previously there was none. The expansion of genomics into mainstream healthcare is bringing many more patients and their families into contact with genomics. This means a much wider range of healthcare professionals such as the Nursing Associate will need knowledge and skills in genomics so as to offer support to families and to help translate genomic advances into better and advanced patient outcomes.

20 Health inequalities

At the point of registration, the Nursing Associate will be able to: understand the factors that may lead to inequalities in health outcomes.

Figure 20.1 Health inequalities.

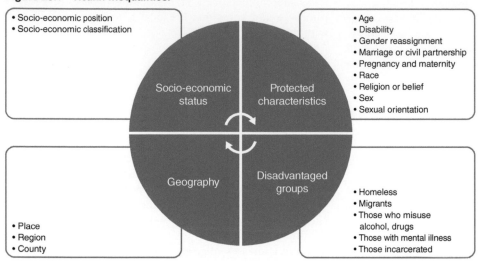

- Socio-economic position
- Socio-economic classification

Socio-economic status

Protected characteristics
- Age
- Disability
- Gender reassignment
- Marriage or civil partnership
- Pregnancy and maternity
- Race
- Religion or belief
- Sex
- Sexual orientation

Geography

Disadvantaged groups

- Place
- Region
- County

- Homeless
- Migrants
- Those who misuse alcohol, drugs
- Those with mental illness
- Those incarcerated

Box 20.1 Some examples of long-term conditions.

- Diabetes
- Cardiovascular (hypertension, angina)
- Chronic respiratory (asthma, chronic obstructive pulmonary disease)
- Chronic neurological (multiple sclerosis, epilepsy)
- Chronic pain (arthritis, osteoarthritis)
- Other long-term conditions (chronic fatigue syndrome, irritable bowel syndrome, cancer)
- Communicable diseases (Human Immunodeficiency Virus, hepatitis B and C)
- Certain mental health disorders (schizophrenia, depression)
- Ongoing impairments in structure (blindness, joint disorders).

Top Tip

Health inequalities are avoidable and unfair differences in the health between groups of people.

There is much evidence that social factors, including education, employment status, level of income, gender and ethnicity have a clear influence on how healthy a person is. Globally, there are wide disparities in the health status of different social groups. The lower an individual's socio-economic position, the higher their risk of poor health. Health inequalities are closely related to the social determinants of health. Understanding these factors can help the Nursing Associate focus on those who experience inequality.

Reducing health inequalities involves giving everyone the same opportunities so they are able to lead a healthy life, regardless of where they live or who they are. People living in the least deprived areas live around 20 years longer in good health than those people in the most deprived areas. Addressing and tackling these inequalities means that more attention has to be given to those who are at greatest risk of poor health if there is to be any impact.

Health inequalities

There are many kinds of health inequality, and the term is used in many ways. Health inequities are systematic differences in the health status of different population groups. These inequities bring with them substantial social and economic costs both to individuals and societies.

Types of inequality

Health inequalities refer to the differences in the status of people's health. The term is also often used to refer to differences in the care that people receive as well as the opportunities that they have to lead healthy lives, both of which can contribute to their health status. Therefore, health inequalities can result in differences in health status (life expectancy and prevalence of health conditions), access to care (the availability of treatments), quality and experience of care (levels of patient satisfaction), behavioural risks to health (smoking rates, alcohol consumption) and wider determinants of health (quality of housing, educational attainment).

Who experiences inequalities?

The differences in health status and the factors that determine it can be experienced by people who are grouped by a range of factors. Often, health inequalities are analysed and addressed by policy across four factors:

- Socio-economic factors (income)
- Geography (region – urban or rural)
- Specific characteristics including those protected characteristics (sex, ethnicity or disability)

- Socially excluded groups (those experiencing homelessness, those who are incarcerated).

See Figure 20.1.

How inequalities are experienced
Life expectancy
A key measure of a population's health status is life expectancy. Inequality in life expectancy is one of the foremost measures of health inequality.

Inequalities in healthy life expectancy
Another key measure of health inequality is how much time people spend in good health throughout their lives, given how crucial good health is to a wider quality of life and people's ability to do the things that they value.

Inequalities in avoidable death
Some deaths can be prevented through preventive interventions or timely health care. Differences in rates of avoidable mortality between population groups reflect differences in people getting the help that they need to address life-threatening health risks and illnesses.

Inequalities in long-term health conditions
One of the major causes of poor quality of life in England are long-term conditions (LTCs) (see Box 20.1). More than 50% of people with a LTC see their health as a barrier to the type or amount of work that they can do, and when a person has three or more conditions this rises to 80%. LTCs can have an indirect impact on health, given the importance of being employed in good-quality work for a person's physical and mental health. See also Chapter 64.

Inequalities in the prevalence of mental ill health
Evidence suggests that inequalities in various types of mental ill health are evident across a range of protected characteristics. People who identify as lesbian, gay, bisexual or transgender (LGBT), for example, experience higher rates of poor mental health than those who do not identify as LGBT.

Inequalities in access to and experience of health services
This refers to the availability of services that are timely, appropriate, sensitive and easy to use. Inequitable access can result in some groups receiving less care relative to their needs, or more inappropriate or suboptimal care, than others, often leading to poorer experiences, outcomes and health status.

21 Early years and childhood: life choices

At the point of registration, the Nursing Associate will be able to: understand the importance of early years and childhood experiences and the possible impact on life choices, mental, physical and behavioural health and well-being.

Figure 21.1 Adverse childhood experiences.

CHILD MALTREATMENT

Verbal abuse   Physical abuse   Sexual abuse

CHILDHOOD HOUSEHOLD INCLUDED

Parental separation | Domestic violence | Mental illness | Alcohol abuse | Drug use | Incarceration

Figure 21.3 Adverse Childhood Experiences – the Life Course (Source: Bellis et al., 2016; Felitti et al., 1988 image credit to Warren Larkin Associates Limited).

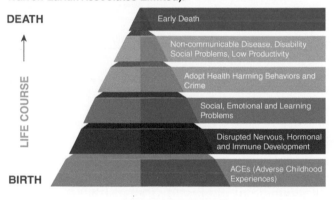

DEATH

LIFE COURSE

BIRTH

Early Death

Non-communicable Disease, Disability Social Problems, Low Productivity

Adopt Health Harming Behaviors and Crime

Social, Emotional and Learning Problems

Disrupted Nervous, Hormonal and Immune Development

ACEs (Adverse Childhood Experiences)

Figure 21.2 Three toxic stress responses (Source: Harvard University, Centre for the Developing Child, 2020).

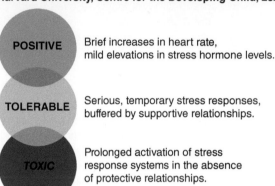

POSITIVE — Brief increases in heart rate, mild elevations in stress hormone levels.

TOLERABLE — Serious, temporary stress responses, buffered by supportive relationships.

TOXIC — Prolonged activation of stress response systems in the absence of protective relationships.

Box 21.1 Impact of number of adverse childhood experiences.

4 times – more likely to be a high-risk drinker
6 times – more likely to have had or caused unintended teenage pregnancy
6 times – more likely to smoke e-cigarettes or tobacco
6 times – more likely to have had sex under the age of 16 years
11 times – more likely to have smoked cannabis
14 times – more likely to have been a victim of violence over the last 12 months
15 times – more likely to have committed violence against another person in the last 12 months
16 times – more likely to have used crack cocaine or heroin
20 times – more likely to have been incarcerated at any point in their lifetime

Top Tip

The future of any society will depend on how it fosters the healthy development of its next generation. Extensive research on the biology of stress shows that healthy development can be overturned by the excessive or prolonged activation of stress response systems in the body and brain.

Adverse childhood experiences

Adverse childhood experiences (ACEs) are an increasing concern nationally and internationally. A growing body of evidence suggests that our experiences during childhood have the potential to affect health throughout the life course. ACEs are not just a concern for healthcare practitioners. Those who have lived unpleasant life experiences in their childhood are more likely to perform poorly in school, more likely to be involved in crime and they are less likely to be a productive member of society.

ACEs are stressful experiences that have occurred during childhood that directly harm a child, for example, sexual or physical abuse, or those that impact the environment in which they are living, such as growing up in a house with domestic violence.

There are three direct and six indirect experiences that have an impact on childhood development (see Figure 21.1). The more adversity that a child experiences, the more likely it is to impact their mental and physical health. Children who are exposed to four or more ACEs are more likely to participate in risk-taking behaviours, find it more difficult to make changes and consequently will have poorer health outcomes

Toxic stress

Children who have experienced stressful and poor-quality childhoods are more likely to adopt health-harming behaviours during their adolescence, which can then lead to mental health illnesses and diseases such as cancer, heart disease and diabetes later in their life. An important part of healthy child development is learning how to cope with adversity. When threatened, our bodies prepare us to respond by increasing the heart rate, blood pressure and stress hormones, such as cortisol. When a young child's stress response systems are stimulated within an environment of caring relationships with adults, these physiological effects are usually buffered and return to baseline. Typically, the result is the development of healthy stress response systems. If the stress response, however, is intense and protracted and uncaring, buffering relationships are unavailable to the child. The outcome can be damaged, weakened systems and brain function, bringing with it lifelong repercussions (see Figure 21.2).

Children growing up with toxic stress may have difficulty in forming healthy and stable relationships. As adults they may also have unstable work histories and they can struggle with finances, family, jobs and depression throughout life, the effects of which may be passed on to their own children.

Consequences of ACEs

Preventing ACEs has the potential to improve health across the whole life course, enhancing individuals' well-being and their productivity while reducing pressures and costs on health, social services, criminal justice and educational systems. Those who experience adverse incidents are more likely to be involved in violence and other antisocial behaviour and to perform more poorly at school.

Preventing or reducing the impact of ACEs can also reduce levels of health-harming behaviours, for example, problem alcohol use, smoking, poor diet and violent behaviour. See Box 21.1, which details the impact that ACEs and the number of these experiences can have on the person.

Physiological changes that occur because of adverse experiences in childhood increase the wear and tear on the body, which in turn increases the risks of premature ill health, for example, cancer, cardiac disease and mental illness. See Figure 21.3.

Preventing ACEs

The childhood years, from the prenatal period up to late adolescence, are the 'building block' years. These years help to set the stage for adult relationships, behaviours, health and social outcomes. ACEs along with their associated harms are preventable. Creating and sustaining safe, stable, nurturing relationships and environments for all children and families can prevent ACEs and help all children to reach their full health and life potential.

The development of cross-governmental approaches and strategies can mitigate the harms of ACEs. ACEs can be prevented by strengthening economic support for families, promoting social norms that protect against violence and adversity, ensure a strong start for children and pave the way for them to reach their full potential. The provision of skill to help parents and younger people handle stress, manage emotions and tackle everyday challenges; early interventions will lessen immediate and long-term harms.

22 Health literacy

Box 22.1   Impact of health literacy on health outcomes.

1 High rates of health literacy in population groups benefit societies.
2 Limited health literacy significantly affects health.
3 Limited health literacy follows a social gradient and can reinforce existing inequalities.
4 Building personal health literacy skills and abilities is a lifelong process.
5 Capacity and competence related to health literacy vary according to context, culture and setting.
6 Responsiveness of health systems facilitates the achievement of positive health outcomes.

Figure 22.1   Health literacy responsiveness of services.

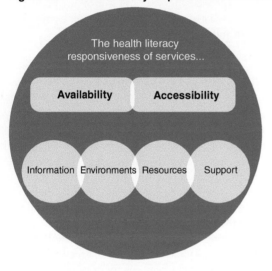

The health literacy responsiveness of services...

Availability   Accessibility

Information   Environments   Resources   Support

Top Tip
Health literacy plays an important role in how well individuals can access health and social care systems and receive quality care.

The Nursing Associate at a Glance, First Edition. Ian Peate.
© 2021 John Wiley & Sons Ltd. Published 2021 by John Wiley & Sons Ltd.

Definition

The World Health Organization (2015) defines health literacy as 'the personal characteristics and social resources needed for individuals and communities to access, understand, appraise and use information and services to make decisions about health'.

Health literacy is a term introduced in the 1970s, and it is becoming more and more important in public health and healthcare. The word *literate* is taken to mean to be 'familiar with literature' or in general terms 'well educated, learned'. Health literacy refers to the degree to which individuals can obtain, process and understand basic health information and the services needed to make appropriate health decisions.

When people have good levels of health literacy, they can improve the skills and confidence needed to make informed decisions about their health and the health of their families, to participate in their care and to effectively navigate healthcare systems.

Health literacy

Emphasis is placed on encouraging better patient participation in their healthcare, particularly with reference to people managing their long-term conditions or promotion of their well-being by those who develop policy. In general, participation implies that patients play more of an active role in their healthcare, including sharing information on their healthcare priorities and taking part in decision-making about their care. Those with low health literacy may find it difficult to participate in their healthcare, resulting in poorer health outcomes. The role of the Nursing Associate, and others, is to provide:

- The right environment
- Information
- Appropriate resources
- Support

All the above approaches are required to ensure that service provision is responding appropriately (see Figure 22.1).

Health literacy contributes to health inequalities because the population groups most at risk of low health literacy are also known to have the poorest health outcomes. Box 22.1 outlines the impact of health literacy on health outcomes. Limited health literacy can also undermine a person's ability to take control of their own health and the conditions that affect their health.

Nutbeam's Health Literacy Model

Nutbeam (2020) offered a health literacy model that is useful in analysing the literacy abilities that are required in various health situations. This model describes three sequential levels of health literacy.

Basic/functional literacy: This encompasses sufficient basic skills in reading and writing to be able to function effectively in everyday situations, broadly compatible with the narrow definition of 'health literacy' referred to above.

Communicative/interactive literacy: This encompasses more advanced cognitive and literacy skills which, together with social skills, can be used to actively participate in everyday activities, to extract information and derive meaning from different forms of communication, and to apply new information to changing circumstances.

Critical literacy: This encompasses more advanced cognitive skills, which, together with social skills, can be applied to critically analyse information, and to use this information to exert greater control over life events and situations.

The three levels (classifications) indicate that the different stages of literacy progressively permit more autonomy and personal empowerment. Progression between levels does not depend only on cognitive development, but also on exposure to different information/messages (communication content and method). In turn, this is influenced by personal responses to such communication, and this is mediated by personal and social skills.

Integrated cross-sector working can promote health literacy with professionals from health and social care services supported by those from other sectors, for example, child and adult education services and the third sector. Employers, communities and families also have a role to play in implementing successful health literacy initiatives.

23 Health screening

At the point of registration, the Nursing Associate will be able to: explain why health screening is important and identify those who are eligible for screening.

Box 23.1   Screening Programmes in England (Public Health England, 2017).

1 Abdominal aortic aneurysm screening
2 Bowel cancer screening
3 Breast cancer screening
4 Cervical screening
5 Diabetic eye screening
6 Foetal anomaly screening
7 Infectious diseases in pregnancy screening
8 Newborn and infant examination programme
9 Newborn blood spot screening
10 Newborn hearing screening
11 Sickle cell and thalassaemia screening.

Table 23.1 Screening and testing (Public Health Action and Support Team, 2017).

	Screening	Diagnostic tests
Purpose	To detect potential disease indicators	To establish presence/absence of disease
Test population	Large numbers of asymptomatic, but potentially at-risk individuals	Symptomatic individuals to establish diagnosis, or asymptomatic individuals with a positive screening test
Test method	Simple, acceptable to patients and staff	May be invasive, expensive but justifiable as necessary to establish diagnosis
Positive end result threshold	Generally chosen towards high sensitivity not to miss potential disease	Chosen towards high specificity (true negatives). More weight given to accuracy and precision than to patient acceptability
Positive result	Essentially indicates suspicion of disease (often used in combination with other risk factors) that warrants confirmation	Result provides a definite diagnosis
Cost to detect potential disease indicators	Cheap; benefits should justify the costs since large numbers of people will need to be screened to identify a small number of potential cases	Higher costs associated with diagnostic test may be justified to establish diagnosis

Top Tip
Screening is designed to identify those people who have the early stages of a disease or an increased chance of developing a disease or condition.

The Nursing Associate at a Glance, First Edition. Ian Peate.

Public health is managed slightly differently in each country of the UK, and this includes public health issues that are associated with population screening.

In England, 11 screening programmes are available (see Box 23.1).

Health screening

Screening is the process of identifying those people who appear healthy but may be at increased risk of a disease or condition. The benefits of screening tests have to outweigh the harm they can cause. A diagnostic test is a test that determines whether a condition is present with 100% accuracy. A screening test, however, looks at the risk of whether a condition is present. It does not offer the person a definite 'yes' or 'no' answer.

Screening is achieved by means of tests, examinations or other procedures that can be applied rapidly and easily to the target population. A screening programme has to include all the core components in the screening process, from inviting the target population to accessing effective treatment for individuals diagnosed with disease. Screening requires a coordinated quality-assured system. The screening provider offers information, further tests and treatment, with the aim of reducing associated problems or complications. The screening programme should do more good than harm, and it has to be provided at an affordable cost.

The Nursing Associate is part of the public health care team. Understanding the key issues regarding screening and their role in improving screening uptake is key to saving lives and improving health and well-being.

Purpose of screening programmes

The aim of screening is to identify people who have the early stages of a disease or to find out if they have an increased chance of developing a disease or condition. The aim of screening includes the following:

- Saving lives by treating disease in their early stages, thus increasing the survival chances of the patient
- Improving the quality of the patient's life through early identification
- Reducing the chance of developing the disease or halting disease progression by permitting the patient to make life changes
- Saving the NHS money by treating in early stages as opposed to later, complicated stages
- Helping meet NHS targets for disease elimination/detection.

Screening and testing

Screening populations is not the same as testing. They may appear the same, but there are differences. Screening is directed towards a specific population and a specific disease. A population refers to people who have been grouped on the basis of a particular characteristic or feature, for example, all those people who have attended a GP surgery with a specific condition, all males aged between 65 and 75 years, or all pregnant women.

During screening, some people being screened may be healthy, well and have no signs or symptoms of the condition that the screening targets. The aim of the screening programmes is to find those people who are at a higher risk, to identify significant health problems before symptoms appear so as to make early treatment available. People in the population are asked questions or offered tests; they are then referred for more accurate tests, and treatment is offered, if needed. Table 23.1 provides an overview of the differences between screening and diagnostic tests.

Population screening

The screening process can be seen as a sieve whereby a large group of people accept the offer of a screening test. The holes in the sieve are a certain size that will catch some people and allow others to pass through. This means they have a low chance of having the condition being screened for, whereas the people left in the sieve have a higher chance of having the condition, and a further investigation is offered to them.

Identification through this process can demonstrate that they have the condition they are being screened for, and the person may need further confirmatory diagnostic tests. At all stages of the screening process, people can make their own choices about:

- Tests
- Treatment
- Advice
- Support.

24 Immunisation and vaccination

At the point of registration, the Nursing Associate will be able to: promote health and prevent ill health by understanding the evidence base for immunisation, vaccination and herd immunity.

Table 24.1 NHS vaccination schedule (NHS, 2019).

Babies under 1 year old	**8 Weeks:** 6-in-1 vaccine, Rotavirus vaccine, MenB **12 weeks:** 6-in-1 vaccine (2nd dose), Pneumococcal (PCV) vaccine, Rotavirus vaccine (2nd dose) **16 weeks:** 6-in-1 vaccine (3rd dose), Rotavirus vaccine, MenB (2nd dose) dose
Children aged 1–15	**1 Year:** Hib/MenC (1st dose), MMR (1st dose), Pneumococcal (PCV) vaccine (2nd dose), MenB (3rd dose) **2 to 10 years:** Flu vaccine (every year) **3 years and 4 months:** MMR (2nd dose), 4-in-1 pre-school booster **12 to 13 years:** HPV vaccine **14 years:** 3-in-1 teenage booster MenACWY
Adults	**65 years:** Pneumococcal (PCV) vaccine **65 years (and every year after):** Flu vaccine **70 years:** Shingles vaccine
Pregnant women	When offered **During flu season:** Flu vaccine **From 16 weeks pregnant:** Whooping cough (pertussis) vaccine

*The COVID-19 vaccine was introduced in the UK in December 2020.

Top Tip

Like any medicine, vaccines can cause mild side effects, for example, low-grade fever, or pain or redness at the injection site. Mild reactions go away within a few days on their own. Severe or long-lasting side effects are extremely rare.

The Nursing Associate at a Glance, First Edition. Ian Peate.
© 2021 John Wiley & Sons Ltd. Published 2021 by John Wiley & Sons Ltd.

Other chapters in this text have made clear that one of the many roles of the Nursing Associate is to promote health and prevent ill health, immunisation and vaccination also have a key role in health and well-being. Effective immunisation and vaccination programmes contribute to enhancing the health of nations.

Immunisation

Immunisation is the process whereby a person is made immune or resistant to an infectious disease, usually by the administration of a vaccine. Vaccines stimulate the body's own immune system, protecting the person against subsequent infection or disease. Immunisation is a proven tool for the control and elimination of life-threatening infectious diseases, preventing millions of deaths each year. It has clearly defined target groups, can be delivered effectively through outreach activities and does not require any major lifestyle change.

Immunisation and public health

One of the most successful public health interventions is immunisation. Immunisation offers protection to children and adults and is saving thousands of lives each year. Healthcare practitioners (and this may include the Nursing Associate) may be required to explain why vaccinations are still so important. Being able to respond and explain can ensure ongoing public and professional confidence and the rapid spread of any vaccine concerns or controversies. Public awareness and confidence in vaccines is quickly shared via electronic and other media. Those providing information must be confident, knowledgeable and up to date.

The immunisation programmes provided in the UK are carefully considered and evidence-based, and for most vaccines, this forms part of an NHS-funded programme. With the ongoing development of new and improved vaccines and the constantly changing epidemiology of infectious diseases, there may be a need to modify vaccine programmes or introduce new ones. See Table 24.1.

Immunity

Immunity is the ability of the human body to protect itself from infectious disease. The defence mechanisms of the body are complex and include innate (non-specific, non-adaptive) mechanisms and acquired (specific, adaptive) systems. Innate or non-specific immunity is present from birth. It includes physical barriers (such as intact skin and mucous membranes), chemical barriers (such as gastric acid, digestive enzymes and bacteriostatic fatty acids of the skin), phagocytic cells and the complement system. Acquired immunity is normally specific to a single organism or to a group of closely related organisms. There are two basic mechanisms for acquiring immunity: active and passive.

Vaccination

Vaccines reduce the risks of getting a disease, working with the body's natural defences to build protection. When a vaccine is given, the immune system responds by:

- Recognising the invading organism, for example, the virus or bacteria.
- Producing antibodies.
- Remembering the disease and how to fight it. If the person is then exposed to the organism in future, the immune system can act quickly before the person becomes unwell.

The vaccine is a safe way to produce an immune response in the body, without causing illness. Once exposed to one or more doses of a vaccine, typically the person remains protected against a disease for years, decades or even a lifetime. Rather than treating a disease after it has occurred, vaccines prevent people from becoming unwell in the first instance.

Herd immunity

Herd immunity is the indirect protection from a contagious infectious disease occurring when a population is immune, whether by vaccination or by immunity developed through previous infection.

This means that even people who are not vaccinated, or in whom the vaccine does not trigger immunity, are protected because people around them who are immune can act as buffers between them and an infected person.

When herd immunity has been established for a while and the ability of the disease to spread has been obstructed, the disease can eventually be eliminated. This is how smallpox was eradicated.

25 Infection, prevention and control

At the point of registration, the Nursing Associate will be able to: protect health through understanding and applying the principles of infection prevention and control, including communicable disease surveillance and antimicrobial stewardship and resistance.

Table 25.1 Personal protective equipment (RCN, 2017).

Disposable gloves	Gloves are not a substitute for hand hygiene and should be used when appropriate. Overuse of gloves is an increasing concern.
Disposable plastic apron	Disposable plastic aprons provide a physical barrier between clothing/skin and prevent contamination and wetting of clothing/uniforms during bathing/washing or equipment cleaning.
Gowns	Impervious (i.e. waterproof) gowns should be used when there is a risk of extensive contamination of blood or body fluids or when local policy dictates their use in certain settings.
Facial mucocutaneous protection	Masks, visors and eye protection should be worn when a procedure is likely to result in blood and body fluids or substances splashing into the eyes, face or mouth – for example, childbirth, trauma or operating theatre environments.

Table 25.2 Health care acquired infection (HCAI) – key facts (WHO, 2016).

Frequency (HAIs)	Globally, on average, 1 in every 10 patients is affected by HAIs. In acute care settings, out of every 100 patients, 7 in developed and 15 in developing countries will get at least one HAI.
Intensive care	In high-income countries, up to 30% of patients are affected by at least one HAI in intensive care units; the frequency in developing countries is at least 2–3 times higher.
Injection safety	Annually there are 16 billion injections administered worldwide, up to 70%of which are given with reused syringes and needles in some developing countries.
Hand hygiene	It is estimated that 61% of health workers do not adhere to recommended hand hygiene practices.
Neonatal care	Amongst babies born in hospital, infections are responsible for 4%–56% of all causes of death occurring in the neonatal period.
Antimicrobial resistance	Patients infected with methicillin-resistant *Staphylococcus aureus* (MRSA) are around 50% more likely to die than those infected with non-resistant strains.

Top Tip

It may seem a strange principle to enunciate as the very first requirement in a Hospital that it should do the sick no harm. Florence Nightingale (1863) *Notes on Hospitals*.

The Nursing Associate at a Glance, First Edition. Ian Peate.
© 2021 John Wiley & Sons Ltd. Published 2021 by John Wiley & Sons Ltd.

When the Nursing Associate employs the principles of infection prevention and control, they are helping to protect health. Infection prevention and control activities include communicable disease surveillance as well as antimicrobial stewardship and resistance.

Infection prevention and control

Infection prevention and control (IPC) is an evidence-based practical approach that prevents patients, Nursing Associates and other health workers from being harmed by avoidable infection. It is key in patient safety and high quality patient care, relevant to every healthcare worker and patient at each and every healthcare interaction. Preventing healthcare-associated infections (HAI) avoids this unnecessary risk and even death, saves money, reduces the spread of antimicrobial resistance and supports high-quality, integrated, people-centred health services.

Principles of infection, prevention and control

Hand hygiene

Hand hygiene describes processes that render the hands of healthcare workers safe (reducing the number of microorganisms acquired through activities involving touching equipment). Hand hygiene includes handwashing, surgical scrub and the use of alcohol gel. The type of hand hygiene performed depends on the type of care that will or has been carried out.

Personal protective equipment

Personal protective equipment (PPE) includes items such as gloves, aprons, masks, goggles or visors. PPE can protect healthcare workers from harm and from risks of infection (see Table 25.1).

Safe handling and disposal of sharps

Sharps include needles, scalpels, stitch cutters, glass ampoules, bone fragments and any sharp instrument. The key hazards of a sharps injury are blood-borne viruses, for example, hepatitis B, hepatitis C and HIV. Staff can be injured by the unsafe or poor practice of others; for example, those who sustain injuries as a result of sharps being inappropriately placed in waste bins. Sharps injuries are preventable.

Safe handling and disposal of waste

Waste that is generated may include sharps, hazardous, offensive, household and pharmaceutical waste. The workplace should have a written policy on waste segregation and disposal providing the Nursing Associate and others with guidance.

Health care acquired infection

An HAI is an infection acquired by a patient during care delivery in a hospital or other healthcare setting that was not present or incubating when the patient was admitted. Visitors, family members and health workers may also be affected by HAIs.

HAIs are mostly caused by microorganisms resistant to one or more commonly used antibiotic. Common HAIs include, urine, chest, blood and wound infections

HAIs can cause unnecessary death. They result in a human and economic burden. Hospital stays are prolonged when a patient has an HAI, and this creates long-term disability and also increases the burden of antimicrobial resistance (AMR). Without regular HAI surveillance as part of an IPC programme, recognising the burden locally and nationally in order to prioritise action would be impossible. See Table 25.2.

HAIs are not limited to just hospitals, and healthcare workers who practice in community settings (including GP surgeries, patients' own homes and care homes) have the same professional and clinical obligations as staff working in hospitals to prevent opportunities for infection from occurring, although the type and level of risk can vary.

Antimicrobial resistance

AMR occurs when microorganisms (for example, bacteria, fungi, viruses and parasites) change when they are exposed to antimicrobial drugs (these include antibiotics, antifungals, antivirals, antimalarials and anthelmintics). Microorganisms that develop AMR are sometimes referred to as 'superbugs'. As a result, medicines become ineffective and infections continue in the body, increasing the risk of transmission to others.

Antibiotic stewardship

The term 'antimicrobial stewardship' is defined as 'an organisational or healthcare-system-wide approach to promoting and monitoring judicious use of antimicrobials to preserve their future effectiveness'.

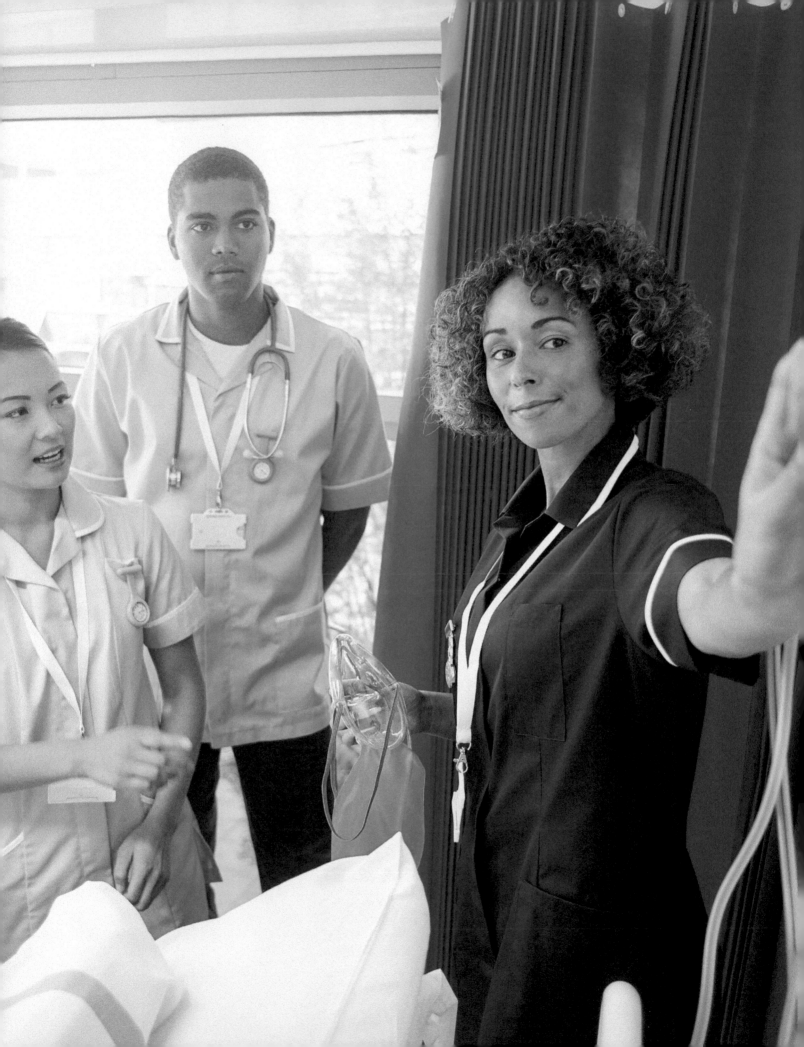

Provide and monitor care

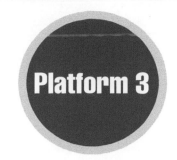

Platform 3

Chapters

26 Human development

At the point of registration, the Nursing Associate will be able to: demonstrate an understanding of human development from conception to death, to enable delivery of person-centred safe and effective care.

Box 26.1 Developmental stages.

- Prenatal
- Infancy
- Early childhood
- Middle childhood
- Adolescence
- Young adulthood
- Middle adulthood
- Late adulthood

Figure 26.1 Life stages (Public Health England, 2019).

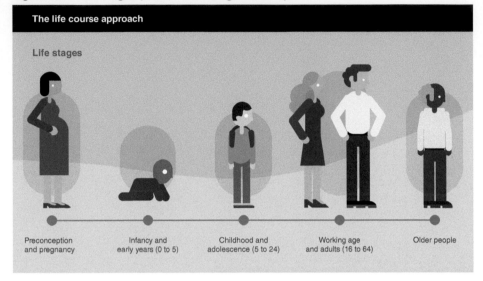

Figure 26.2 Influencing factors.

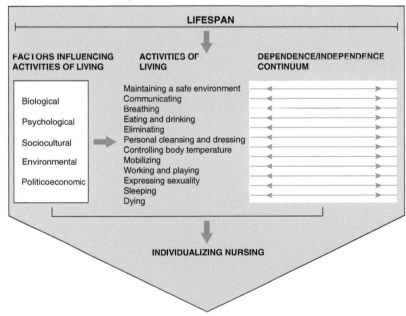

Top Tip

Health is the result of many transactions that occur between genetic, biological, behavioural, social and economic contexts; they change as an individual develops over time.

The Nursing Associate at a Glance, First Edition. Ian Peate.
© 2021 John Wiley & Sons Ltd. Published 2021 by John Wiley & Sons Ltd.

The human develops from conception to death in a number of ways with developmental indicators related to their physical and cognitive milestones and their psychosocial development.

A person's physical and emotional development is cumulative; that is, it happens over time. Our experiences during each stage of the lifespan have an impact on how subsequent stages will be experienced; these can be good or bad. Experiences, exposures and environments impact a person throughout their life. The Nursing Associate needs to understand the various stages of development as this can help them as they offer person-centred care in a safe and effective way.

The process of human development can be considered from multiple phases; for example, see Box 26.1 and Figure 26.1. These various stages should never be considered as individual silos.

The lifespan

This can be seen as a continuum from conception to death. As an individual moves along the lifespan there is continuous change, growth and development. However, it should be noted this is not the same for everyone, and the speed at which a person develops is also not the same for everyone. Generally, it could be suggested that younger people and older people may need more help, whilst young and middle-aged adults may need less help.

It is important to note that the lifespan cannot be considered in insolation. The Nursing Associate must take other factors into account (see Figure 26.2).

Prenatal

The unborn child will be impacted by the safety and health of its life in the uterus or by any conditions that risk this. The emotional experiences of the mother are likely to affect the child's infancy as well.

Infancy

The first decisive human relationship which a person has, already established in the prenatal stage, is with their mother. A child may be expected to develop feelings of security. Erikson (1963) suggests that the infant begins to experience a sense of comfort even whilst becoming aware of its dependence on others. Trust and comfort are undeniably essential to the healthy development of the child; when absent, this can have emotionally devastating effects on the development of the individual's ego orientation.

Early and middle childhood

How a child develops in early childhood is impacted by environmental surroundings as well as by individual capabilities. It is possible to facilitate the proper socialisation of a child, enabling the appropriate development of physical, emotional and cognitive abilities. What happens at home plays a key role in shaping the early capabilities of children. The child usually learns to walk, talk and feed themselves, developing finer motor skills. Self-esteem and autonomy develop, and during middle childhood, the child begins to develop an understanding of moral structures, influenced by a number of factors.

Adolescence

At this point, the individual is able to observe the value of actions and decisions as opposed to viewing them in the form of personal repercussions, leading to a sense of the world as separate from themselves. During this stage, significant physical, psychological and social changes take place. Childhood passes through adolescence and into early adulthood.

Young and middle adulthood

During this stage, commitments are made with others rather than with parents or family. The moral compass is developed and applied where dilemmas and internal conflicts are encountered. This is a period accompanied by a growing awareness of personal identity along with a clearer insight into the ethical implications of actions taken. If this stage of development is distorted, a deficit in all the following stages could result. During middle adulthood, the person establishes themselves professionally, financially and romantically. This stage marks a change for the adult to experience a sense of meaning independent of this critical role as a parent, nurturer and provider.

Late adulthood

Older adults often reflect on their lives, usually with happiness and contentment, feeling fulfilled with a sense that life has meaning and the person has made a contribution to life, something that Erikson refers to as integrity.

58

Platform 3 Provide and monitor care

27 Anatomy and physiology

At the point of registration, the Nursing Associate will be able to: demonstrate and apply knowledge of body systems and homeostasis, human anatomy and physiology, biology, genomics, pharmacology, social and behavioural sciences when delivering care.

Figure 27.1   Levels of organisation of the body.

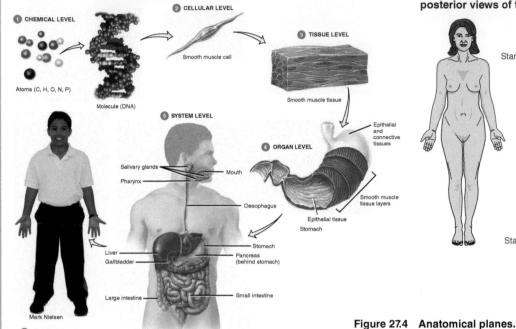

Figure 27.2   Anatomical position: anterior and posterior views of the body.

Standing erect, facing observer

Palms facing forward

Standing flat on feet

Figure 27.4   Anatomical planes.

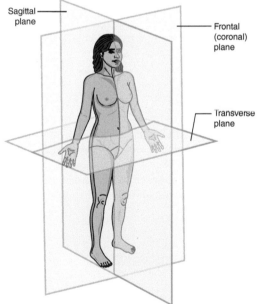

Sagittal plane

Frontal (coronal) plane

Transverse plane

Figure 27.3   Anatomical position.

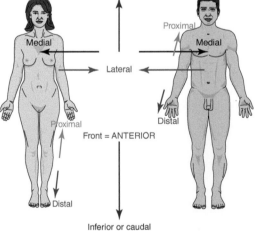

Cephalad, Cranial or Superior

Proximal

Medial

Medial

Lateral

Proximal

Distal

Front = ANTERIOR

Distal

Inferior or caudal

Top Tip

To provide expert patient care, a broad understanding of anatomy and physiology is just as important as compassion, communication, courage or any of the other 6Cs.

The Nursing Associate at a Glance, First Edition. Ian Peate.
© 2021 John Wiley & Sons Ltd. Published 2021 by John Wiley & Sons Ltd.

Many chapters in this text encourage the Nursing Associate to demonstrate and apply their knowledge of human anatomy and physiology, biology, genomics (see Chapter 19), pharmacology (see Chapters 40–42), social and behavioural sciences (see, for example, Chapter 18) when offering care to people.

Anatomy and Physiology

The Nursing Associate requires a range of expert skills and knowledge to care successfully for patients.

'Anatomy and Physiology' is a key course in any programme of study that any nursing and healthcare student must undertake in order to be admitted to the professional register. Understanding anatomy and physiology is essential as a perquisite for the foundation of the work that the Nursing Associate performs each day. Successful care delivery demands insight and understanding of the various body systems, homeostasis, genomics, pharmacology and social and behavioural sciences when delivering care. The Nursing Associate is required to apply this understanding to care.

Anatomy and physiology describe the structure and function of the body. Individual body systems act together so as to operate effectively. Both of these terms are interlinked; understanding where the various parts of the body are located can help the Nursing Associate also understand how they function. Another term, *pathology*, relates to the study of disease in the body.

Body systems

The human body is as beautiful on the inside as it is on the outside; it is a marvel. The body is a complicated structure, originating from a number of different cell types that form tissues, organs and systems. A variety of intricate processes are involved in the effective functioning of the numerous body systems. The level of organisation of the body is found in Figure 27.1.

Homeostasis

Homoeostasis is seen as the regulation of the body's internal environment, providing a level of consistency that is maintained for the cells and organs of the body to function in an effective way. Homeostatic mechanisms work in such a way that the body is able to manage with any external changes and in so doing secures stability. When homeostatic mechanisms fail and there is no, or a poor, response to the impact of external changes, this is when 'dis–ease' (disease) occurs. Disease is a breakdown or an upset in the body's ability to self-regulate.

Anatomical terminology

Science, especially nursing and medicine, is filled with Latin and Greek terminologies. Latin names are used for every part of the body, and Greek terms are common as the Greeks are said to be the founders of modern medicine.

The body map

Learning anatomical terminology is akin to learning a new language; this can help you talk confidently about the body. The anatomical directional terms and the body planes present a universally recognised language of anatomy. You will need to have an understanding of key or directional terminology in you vocabulary to give a precise description as you or others refer to the precise location of a body part or structure.

All parts of the body are described in relation to other body parts. A standardised body position known as the anatomical position is used in anatomical terminology. An anatomical position is established from an imaginary central line that runs down the centre or mid-line of the body. When in this position the body is erect and faces forwards, with the arms to the side, palms face forwards with the thumbs to the side, the feet are slightly apart and the toes point forwards (see Figure 27.2).

Understanding directional terms and the position of the various structures is also required (see Figure 27.3).

Anatomical planes of the body

A plane is an imaginary two-dimensional surface passing through the body. There are three planes, generally referred to in anatomy and healthcare (see Figure 27.4).

Anatomical regions of the body

The body is divided up into regions, like a map. The anatomical regions of the body refer to a particular area/region of the body. This helps in compartmentalisation. The body is divided into the:

- Head and neck
- Trunk (thorax and abdomen)
- Upper limbs (arms)
- Lower limbs (legs)

In order to communicate safely with other healthcare professionals, it is essential that the language used is consistent so as to reduce any risk of confusion. Learning the language requires practice.

28 Commonly encountered conditions when delivering care

At the point of registration, the Nursing Associate will be able to: recognise and apply knowledge of commonly encountered mental, physical, behavioural and cognitive health conditions when delivering care.

Table 28.1 Spheres of practice.

Field	Examples of spheres of practice
Child	Hospitals Day care centres Child health clinics Child's own home Community
Learning disabilities	People's homes Education Workplaces Residential and community centres Hospitals Mental health settings Prisons
Mental health	Psychiatric intensive care unit Psychiatric ward Outpatient unit Specialist unit dealing with eating disorders. GP surgery Prisons Community healthcare centre Residential centre Patients' own homes
Adult	Hospital wards, outpatient units or specialist departments Patient's home, Clinics GP surgery Walk-in centres Nursing homes. Prisons The police/justice system Voluntary or private sector

Figure 28.1 The interrelated elements affecting people's physical health (Nursing, Midwifery and Allied Health Professions Policy Unit, 2016).

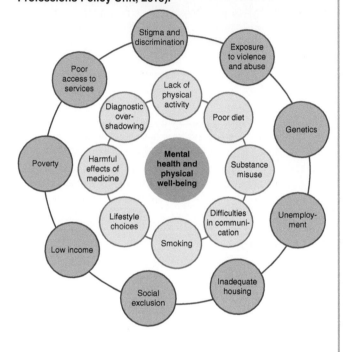

Top Tip

Physical health + mental health = the whole package.

The Nursing Associate, in England, plays a stand-alone role, working with people of all ages and in a variety of settings in health and social care. The role contributes to the core work of nursing across all four fields of nursing (see Table 28.1). This chapter will focus on improving the physical health of people with mental health problems. One in four people will experience a mental health problem at some point in their lives

Parity of esteem

Parity of esteem refers to equal access to effective care and treatment, equal efforts to enhance the quality of care, equal standing within healthcare education and practice, equally high aspirations for those who use services and equal status when measuring health outcomes. However, in achieving parity, this demands action and commitment at multiple levels and requires input from multiple agencies but, most of all the input of those who use services is paramount. The principle 'parity of esteem', which means mental health must be given the same priority as physical health, was protected in law by the Health and Social Care Act 2012.

When there is parity of esteem, mental health and physical health needs will be given the same priority and value, ensuring that people with mental health problems will have equal access to care and treatment. It is an absolute must for health and social care staff to offer the same levels of dignity and respect as well as the same quality of physical healthcare as those offered to people without a mental health illness.

Mortality gap

People who have a serious mental illness are more likely to die 15–20 years before the rest of the general population. This is known as the mortality gap. There are a number of reasons why this mortality gap exists:

- Discrimination
- Stigma
- Poor life chances
- Poor physical health
- Lifestyle choices
- The use of long-term medication
- The way in which mental health services are structured.

The mortality gap is primarily due to physical health problems that often go undiagnosed or are not managed efficiently and life-style factors that can negatively affect the person's physical health. See Figure 28.1 on the interrelated elements affecting people's physical health.

In addressing the discrimination and inequality that people with mental health illness experience, the Nursing Associate and others must acknowledge that that those with mental health illness dying 20 years before the rest of the general population is totally unacceptable. Action has to be taken to improve the quality of life and life expectancy of this population with regard to how their mental health is treated and improved and how their physical health needs are given consideration by mental health professionals (for example, through a reduction in the use of antipsychotic medication).

Improved understanding

Nursing Associates and others who work outside the mental health setting need an improved understanding and the appropriate knowledge and skills to recognise those factors involved in, and the impact of, poor physical health in this patient population. This includes their own role as they work to reduce the unacceptable mortality gap. It is essential to acknowledge the interdependence of good physical and mental health.

Mental healthcare should not be seen as a separate component of care delivery; physical health and mental health are interdependent. In order to care holistically and treat an individual, the Nursing Associate is required to consider the whole person. The mutual impacts of physical ill health and mental ill health have to be addressed as a package.

It is essential that we all enjoy good mental health. A holistic approach to managing mental and physical health is required. Physical and mental health are inseparable, and it is detrimental to an individual's overall well-being to regard these important components as two separate entities. It has been stated that there is evidence that having a long-term mental health condition can be a significant risk factor for the development of physical ill health. On the other hand, long-term physical health conditions can lead to people experiencing poor mental health.

29 # Pre-procedure information giving

At the point of registration, the Nursing Associate will be able to: demonstrate the knowledge, communication and relationship management skills required to provide people, families and carers with accurate information that meets their needs before, during and after a range of interventions.

Table 29.1 Ideas, concerns and expectations (ICE).

Component	Discussion
Ideas	What do you think is causing the problem? Do you have any ideas about what might be going on? It would be helpful to hear what you think might be going on here; you have obviously given this a lot of thought. What do you think might be happening?" What might be your best guess as to what is causing this? Are there any ideas that you have as to what might be going on at the moment?
Concerns	Explain to me your biggest concern regarding what this might be? Do you have any concerns about this being anything in particular? What is the worst thing you were thinking it might be? What is your number one concern regarding this problem right now?
Explanation	What were you hoping we would be able to do for you today? What do you think might be the best plan of action? What were you anticipating would happen today? Do you have any thoughts on the best ways we could tackle the issue?

Box 29.1   Producing patient information.

- Make the text accessible to a wide audience, use short sentences with no more than 15 to 20 words long. Write in lowercase letters where possible, and use a minimum font size of 12.
- Use present and active tenses such as 'your appointment is on . . .' as opposed to 'your appointment has been made for . . .'
- The appearance of the text is important: white space makes information easier to read. Use small blocks of text: a question-and-answer format or bullet points are effective ways of dividing up blocks of text.
- Use a large bold font to emphasise text (uppercase letters, italics and underlining should not be used).
- Labelled diagrams and pictures can illustrate content. Avoid using clip art. Images and pictures from the NHS photo library can create a more professional finish.

Top Tip

When information is unclear, patients and carers can experience a great deal of anxiety. This can also have a negative impact on the patient experience.

The Nursing Associate at a Glance, First Edition. Ian Peate.
© 2021 John Wiley & Sons Ltd. Published 2021 by John Wiley & Sons Ltd.

nterventions in this context are seen any investigation, procedure or treatment offered to a person.

Information giving

The process of giving information to patients and their families (where appropriate) requires the Nursing Associate to consider a number of factors. This is an important activity in the fields of health and social care. Several factors can affect a patient's response to the information received. Resources and strategies should be implemented and effectiveness assessed when giving people information.

The provision of information is central to a number of roles that the Nursing Associate undertakes. The need for Nursing Associates and other health professionals to help people access high-quality information and provide information to patients effectively is a key feature of the Nursing and Midwifery Council (NMC) Code and other UK policy requirements.

It may become necessary to give people information or provide an explanation regarding, for example:

- The administration of a suppository
- Explaining how to use an inhaler
- Explaining a treatment plan or a new approach to that person's care
- Lifestyle advice to help the patient stop smoking.

The Nursing Associate needs to know how to communicate effectively and also to understand that communicating in the clinical or care setting requires preparation and that an individual/tailored approach is required.

When information is imparted in an effective manner, patients will be well informed and have a clearer understanding when making decisions concerning their care, any investigations and other procedures. The Nursing Associate–patient relationship will also be enhanced, which can reduce patient (and carer) anxiety. A positive Nursing Associate–patient relationship has the potential to strength the bond between the Nursing Associate and patient and lead to enhanced patient outcomes.

Ideas, concerns and expectations (ICE)

A key element of information giving involves the Nursing Associate asking a patient about their ideas, concerns and expectations (referred to as ICE). Using this approach can help the Nursing Associate develop their communication and relationship management skills. Asking about a patient's ideas, concerns and expectations can help in gaining insight into how a patient currently understands and feels about their situation and what it is that they may be concerned about. Table 29.1 outlines some of the ways in which ICE can be used. When people provide answers or offer comments in response to ICE, the Nursing Associate can engage in a more meaningful and focussed manner. The information imparted, for example, prior to a procedure or investigation can be tailored to meet the needs of the patient.

Giving information

When patients are anxious or worried about their condition, treatment or procedure, it can be difficult to retain information and difficult to decide which information is reliable when faced with the plethora of online resources (this was particularly apparent during the COVID-19 pandemic). Therefore, having clear written information that patients can go back to and re-read is vital. Information leaflets are only one type of information the Nursing Associate can provide. This approach is only intended to back up and reinforce verbal information and discussion; they are not a substitute.

Information leaflets

Always write from the patient's point of view, and always assume you have only a little knowledge of the subject. Try and imagine yourself in the patient's shoes. If you were a patient, what would you want to know? Use everyday language, do not be patronising and avoid jargon and acronyms. Use patient-friendly text using personal pronouns, for example, 'we' and 'you'. If it is difficult to avoid using medical terminology, explain what each term means. The information should be complementary to other information – letters and leaflets – and be relevant to individuals. Reinforce any information patients have been told. Explain instructions; for example, why a patient should not eat for six hours. Provide facts about risks, side effects and benefits; this can help people make decisions. Signpost people to other information, support and resources available. Where possible, give the name of an individual they can contact, such as a named nurse. Ensure the information is up to date; provide the most recent practice and latest phone numbers. Let people know if the information is available in other formats.

Box 29.1 provides further information on the use and design of information leaflets.

Shared decision-making

At the point of registration, the Nursing Associate will be able to: work in partnership with people, to encourage shared decision-making, in order to support individuals, their families and carers to manage their own care when appropriate.

Box 30.1 Benefits of shared decision-making.

- Those receiving and those delivering care can understand what is important to the other person.
- People feel supported and empowered to make informed choices, and shared decisions about care are taken.
- Nursing Associates, health and social care professionals can tailor the care or treatment to the needs of the individual.

Figure 30.1 Shared decision-making.

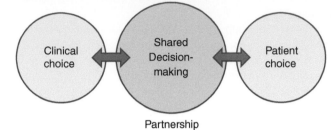

Box 30.2 Some examples of when and where shared decision-making is appropriate.

- Any case where there is more than one reasonable course of action and the decision will involve trade-offs such as length of life versus quality of life
- Where there is uncertainty or unclear evidence for one option over another
- Where options have different inherent risks or benefits or where personal values are important in improving the decision.

Top Tip
People want to be more involved in decisions about their health and care.

The Nursing Associate at a Glance, First Edition. Ian Peate.
© 2021 John Wiley & Sons Ltd. Published 2021 by John Wiley & Sons Ltd.

Providing information and giving people facts about risks, side effects and benefits can help people make decisions. The Nursing and Midwifery Council (NMC) Code requires the Nursing Associate to listen to people and to respond to preferences and concerns. They must encourage and empower people to share in decisions about their treatment and care. Respect must be given to how much people want to be involved in decisions about their own health, well-being and care.

The Nursing Associate must adhere to all relevant laws about mental capacity, ensuring that the rights and best interests of those who lack capacity remain at the centre of the decision-making process.

Personalised care

Personalised care means that people have choice and control over the way their care is planned and delivered. It is based on 'what matters' to them and their individual strengths and needs. Personalised care makes the most of the expertise, capacity and potential of people, families and communities in delivering better outcomes and experiences adopting a whole-system approach.

Shared decision-making

Shared decision-making occurs when health professionals work together to support individuals, their families and carers to manage their own care, when this is appropriate (see Figure 30.1). This places people at the centre of decisions regarding their own treatment and care. It is important that:

- Care or treatment options are fully explored, as well as their risks and benefits
- Different choices available are discussed with the patient
- A decision is reached together with a health and social care professional

The benefits of shared decision-making are outlined in Box 30.1.

Shared decision-making requires skill from professionals and most importantly a commitment to involve patients in decisions about their care. It also requires health and care professionals (including Nursing Associates) to recognise that patients, especially those with lower levels of health literacy, may need support to take a more active partnership role with their care professional. Two sources of expertise are required:

1 The health professional as an expert on the effectiveness, probable benefits and potential harms of treatment options
2 The patient as an expert on themselves, their social circumstances, their attitudes to illness and risk, their values and preferences.

Where there is more than one option in decision-making, the values and preferences of the person, for example, their attitude to risk, can be just as important as the clinical evidence in choosing the option that is to be followed.

Shared decision-making empowers patients to align their preferences with clinically valid treatment options. It does not mean, however, that people can choose clinical treatments that have no evidence base.

Both parties have to be willing to share information and accept shared responsibility for joint decision-making. For some, this may be only a subtle change of practice, but for others and for patients, it could feel like a dramatic one.

Whilst shared decision-making is a key tenet of modern healthcare, far too often it is still not fully practised by clinicians or experienced by patients.

There may be a disconnect between what a clinician thinks they are doing and what a patient thinks that clinicians are doing.

Shared decision-making: care settings

Shared decision-making is appropriate in nearly every situation in community, primary and secondary care where a care decision has to be made, and that decision is said to be 'preference sensitive'.

See Box 30.2 for some examples of when and where shared decision-making is appropriate. Even in some accident and emergency settings, for example chest pain and stroke, it is appropriate to use shared decision-making.

31 Escalating concerns

At the point of registration, the Nursing Associate will be able to: Demonstrate and apply an understanding of how and when to escalate to the appropriate professional for expert help and advice.

Box 31.1 Physiological measurements.

1. Physiological observations should be recorded at the time of admission or initial assessment.
2. A clearly written monitoring plan should detail which physiological observations should be taken and how often.
3. Observations should be carried out by staff trained to undertake these procedures and who appreciate their clinical meaning.
4. Regular assessment of staff taking observations should be done, so as to define competency standards.
5. At a minimum, patient observations should include:
   - Heart rate
   - Respiratory rate
   - Blood pressure
   - Level of consciousness
   - Oxygen saturation including percentage/flow rate of administered oxygen therapy
   - Temperature
   - State of hydration
6. In certain situations, additional monitoring will be required, such as biochemical analysis (for example, blood glucose or lactate) or assessment of pain.

Table 31.1 SBAR.

Situation
- Identify yourself and the site/unit you are calling from.
- Identify the patient by name and the reason for your communication.
- Describe your concern.

Background
- Give the patient's reason for admission.
- Explain significant medical history.
- Inform the receiver of the patient's background: admitting diagnosis, date of admission, previous procedures, current medications, known allergies, relevant laboratory results and other diagnostic results.

Assessment
- Vital signs.
- Glasgow Coma Score.
- Clinical impressions, concerns.

Recommendation
- Explain what you need – be specific about request and time frame.
- Make suggestions.
- Clarify expectations.

Table 31.2 RSVP.

Reason
- State the identity of the caller.
- Check you are speaking to the correct person.
- State the patient's name and location.
- State the reason for the call.

Story
- State background information about the patient.
- Reason for admission.
- State relevant past medical history.
- State the patient's resuscitation status.

Vital Signs
- Temperature.
- Pulse rate and rhythm.
- Blood pressure.
- Breathing rate, conscious level, mental state, capillary refill time, sweating, SaO_2, FiO_2, urine output, NEWS2 score.

Plan
- My plan is . . . or What is your plan?
- Say what is required from the receiver of the call.

Top Tip

Communication failures are a prime cause of patient safety incidents.

The Nursing Associate at a Glance, First Edition. Ian Peate.
© 2021 John Wiley & Sons Ltd. Published 2021 by John Wiley & Sons Ltd.

Chapter 5 of this text considers the role of the Nursing Associate, the demands of professional practice and the need to be able to demonstrate how to recognise signs of vulnerability and to take action required to minimise risks to health and well-being. Chapter 12 highlights the need to recognise and report any factors that may adversely impact safe and effective care provision. This chapter will focus on the need for the Nursing Associate to demonstrate and apply an understanding of how and when to escalate to the appropriate professional for expert help and advice with regard to clinical findings. The Nursing Associate must understand the various roles and functions of members of the multidisciplinary team in order to make appropriate referrals.

The value of the Nursing Associate and other staffs' ability to recognise and respond to deterioration in a patient's condition, tackle adverse events and promote patient safety should not be understated (see also Chapter 35). The recognition and management of the deteriorating patient is complex and multidimensional. As the inpatient population becomes older and sicker with more complex care needs, patient acuity will continue to increase in hospital wards. The provision of education and updating must be in place to enhance the ability to recognise and respond to patient deterioration.

The deteriorating patient

A deteriorating patient can be described as one who moves from one clinical state to a worse clinical state. This increases their individual risk of morbidity, including organ dysfunction, prolonged hospital stay, disability or death. Deterioration in an acutely ill patient's condition can happen quickly and have catastrophic effects. Therefore, observations have to be seen as a fundamental rather than a basic task.

Measurement, documentation and reporting

Measurement, documentation and reporting of physiological observations are fundamental in order to identify a patient's health status (see Box 31.1). These observations provide a baseline that makes it possible to identify clinical deterioration early. Within all healthcare environments, the monitoring, measurement, interpretation and prompt response to physiological observations is one of the core roles undertaken by Nursing Associates and other appropriately prepared staff.

If observations are not recorded and if abnormal observations are not acted upon and communicated effectively, then recognition of the deteriorating patient could be delayed.

A 'track and trigger' system, for example, the National Early Warning Score (NEWS2) uses an aggregated weighted scoring system for each of the core physiological elements of patient observation. The cumulative total of the sub-scores provides an indication of the patient's overall clinical health status at that time, and it can therefore act as a trigger for taking appropriate intervention. When deterioration is detected, local escalation policies and procedures should be initiated, and these should describe the specific clinical intervention(s) that should be taken, empowering the Nursing Associate to escalate their concerns according to policy and adhering to the tenets of the Nursing and Midwifery Council (NMC) Code.

SBAR

Serious clinical errors are very often related to inadequate verbal and written communication. There are some important barriers to communication that occur across different disciplines and levels of staff. These barriers include hierarchy, gender, ethnic background and differences in communication styles between disciplines and individuals. In teams where standard communication structures are in place, for example, SBAR communication, patient safety is enhanced (see Table 31.1).

RSVP

The RSVP system is easy to remember in an emergency and includes the essential information that would enable an experienced clinician to respond appropriately to a call for help from staff. The use of such a structured call for help has the potential to improve patient safety (see Table 31.2).

One of the problems that prevents the deteriorating hospital patient getting prompt and effective treatment is an ineffective call for help from staff who have identified that the patient is acutely unwell. This may because different disciplines communicate in different ways, with the call lacking structure as a result.

32 Dignity and comfort

At the point of registration, the Nursing Associate will be able to: demonstrate and apply an understanding of how people's needs for safety, dignity, privacy, comfort and sleep can be met.

Figure 32.1 The Dignity Challenge.

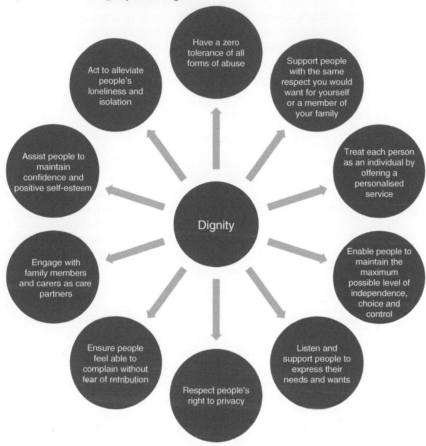

Table 32.1 Appropriate sleep duration for specific age groups (National Sleep Foundation, 2015).

Newborn (0 to 3 months)	14 to 17 hours
Infants (4 to 11 months)	12 to 15 hours
Toddlers (1 to 2 years)	11 to 14 hours
Pre-school (3 to 5 years)	10 to 13 hours
School-age children (6 to 13 years)	9 to 11 hours
Teenagers (14 to 17 years)	8 to 10 hours
Adults (18 to 64 years)	7 to 9 hours
Older adults (over 65 years)	7 to 8 hours

Top Tip

To cure sometimes; to relieve often; to comfort always.
Hippocrates

The Nursing Associate at a Glance, First Edition. Ian Peate.
© 2021 John Wiley & Sons Ltd. Published 2021 by John Wiley & Sons Ltd.

Patient safety

Promoting patient safety and person-centred care are inseparable. Patient safety is concerned with a range of circumstances, situations and occurrences that have the potential to put patients at risk. It may not be one issue that results in a problem; a combination of factors could be at play.

Patient safety is concerned with maximising the things that go right and minimising the things that go wrong. It is key to the NHS' definition of quality in healthcare, and sits alongside effectiveness and patient experience.

Dignity and privacy

There are some people who find accessing health and social care a very undignified experience. As matter of routine (for staff), people are asked to remove their clothing, they are palpated, blood is taken from them and intravenous injections and infusions given to them and investigations allow us peer inside their bodies and to photograph them (X-rays, scans, ultrasounds). We ask people to reveal intimate details (to complete strangers). We ask about things that are very private, how much a person smokes, what they smoke, when they consume alcohol, how much of it and we enquire about their toilet habits. We take their clothes away from them and offer them instead a one-size-fits-all hospital gown. Patients leave the security and comfort of their own homes; they are now visitors in a building they know little about in close proximity to others they have not chosen to be so close to, in a four-bedded ward with people often hearing all that is said about them and others.

Dignity in care is an important concern for patients who seek care and treatment. The Nursing Associate is required to demonstrate their commitment to maintaining patient privacy and dignity. When people are ill, anxious and scared, they look for care, rest and comfort in surroundings where they feel safe, knowing that staff are doing all they can to preserve and promote privacy and dignity. Staff in health and social care organisations must respect patients' rights to privacy and dignity. Privacy refers to freedom from intrusion and encompasses all information and practice that is personal or sensitive. Dignity means being worthy of respect, and the assurance that one's values, beliefs and personal relationships will be respected. The dignified care offered to patients applies to all patients, regardless of their age, gender, ethnicity, social or cultural circumstances, their psychological or physical requirements.

The Dignity in Care campaign aims to put dignity and respect at the heart of UK care services. See Figure 32.1 on the ten-point dignity challenge.

Comfort

Feeling comfortable in or out of bed is important for everyone; it allows us to feel rested and revitalised. In certain settings, it is also a requirement of nursing care when the patient is required to either remain in bed for extended periods of time due to their clinical condition or individual ability.

Comfort is an important nursing issue; it is a fundamental requirement in all aspects of life and is an indispensable component of holistic nursing care. Patients who are comfortable will recover and rehabilitate quicker, manage better or die more peacefully than those who are uncomfortable.

Nursing Associates are required to possess and demonstrate skills in promoting comfort. When patients are in bed, for example, this includes positioning utilising pressure-relieving techniques. See also Chapter 37.

Sleep

Sleep is a complex process that many of us take for granted. The sleep–wake cycle in humans is fundamentally regulated by two significant physiological processes, homeostasis and the endogenous circadian cycle. Homoeostasis encompasses the maintenance of an internal state of equilibrium and stability within the body. The circadian cycle is a complex process that involves among other integrated process the synthesis and release of melatonin by the pineal gland when exposed to darkness.

Sleep deprivation can have a negative impact on a person's health and well-being, in and out of hospital settings. There multiple are interrelated causes of sleep deprivation; some are psychological, some physical and some social.

Multiple pathologies can impact the physical, psychological and social well-being of those who are sleep deprived. The consequences of poor-quality sleep are diverse, involving reduced cognitive ability, mood, decision-making, stress, depression and limited task performance. Poor-quality sleep can result in impaired immunity, cardiovascular and respiratory problems, hormonal changes and urological disease (Table 32.1 outlines appropriate sleep durations for specific groups).

33 Nutrition and hydration

At the point of registration, the Nursing Associate will be able to: demonstrate the knowledge, skills and ability required to meet people's needs related to nutrition, hydration and bladder and bowel health.

Box 33.1 Ascertaining normal eating habits.

- Usual ability to manage independently
- Amount of assistance required
- Food allergies
- Dietary preferences
- Special diets to meet medical or cultural requirements
- Oral health
- Physical difficulties that may affect the ability to eat and drink

Box 33.2 Some signs of dysphagia.

- Coughing when eating a meal
- Regurgitating food
- Food and secretions leaking from the mouth during eating
- Complaining of food sticking and not going down into the stomach
- A wet voice
- Excessive saliva

Box 33.3 Some effects of dehydration.

- Thirst
- Feeling dizzy/light-headed
- Sleepiness/tiredness
- Dry, sticky mouth
- Headache
- Passing small amounts of dark, concentrated urine
- Hypotension
- Tachycardia

Box 33.4 Monitoring hydration.

- Recording input/output where appropriate
- Weighing
- Blood testing
- Physical assessment
- Ask the person if they are thirsty
- Observe oral mucosa
- Blood pressure monitoring

Box 33.5 Some complications of dehydration.

- Constipation
- Infections
- Delayed wound healing
- Delirium
- Falls
- Acute kidney injury
- Death

Box 33.6 Encouraging hydration.

- 2.5 litres of fluid a day is recommended unless there are clinical considerations
- Encourage people to drink small amounts throughout the day and to have more at meal times or with medication
- Offer appropriate choices of drinks
- Ensure that clean, fresh water is accessible
- Where appropriate, encourage family and carer to assist with feeding and drinking
- Provide appropriate aids

Box 33.7 Factors to consider with regard to bowel and bladder health.

- How often the person goes to the toilet to urinate and defaecate and whether this is a change to their normal routine
- Current or previous medical history
- Possibility of physical or sexual abuse, including female genital mutilation
- A rough approximation of the amount of urine passed
- Visual description of the faeces (usually based on Bristol Stool Chart)
- If there is leakage, whether it is urine or faeces
- Information about diet and fluid intake
- Any medications being taken (prescribed and over the counter)
- Lifestyle factors, use of recreational drugs, alcohol, smoking and weight
- Ability – for example, whether the person can feed, dress and bathe on their own
- Mobility – physical or environmental factors
- Does the person recognise the need to go to the toilet or do they forget where the toilet is (capacity)?

Top Tip

There are certain groups of people who are at higher risk of malnutrition, such as those living with chronic conditions, those with mental health needs and those who are approaching the end of life.

Good nutritional care is vital to well-being and health. There are times when people, whatever their age, will be in need of assistance with eating and drinking. Those with malnutrition will have a deficit of vitamins, protein, minerals and energy; this impacts health and well-being. There are a number of complications associated with malnutrition, including poor wound healing, breakdown of the skin, increased risk of developing sepsis and hospital-acquired infections, for example, chest and urinary tract infections. High-quality patient care means that adequate nutrition and hydration are given high priority. The Nursing Associate has to possess the knowledge and skills required to help people with their nutrition, hydration and bladder and bowel health

Malnutrition

Nutritional support in adults has important implications in health and social care settings. When a person is malnourished, basic health and social care outcomes are significantly affected. Malnutrition should be seen as an important patient safety issue. It continues to be under-detected and undertreated, bringing with it fatal consequences. Malnutrition is defined as a state in which there is a deficiency of nutrients such as energy, protein, vitamins or minerals that results in measurable effects on body structure, function or clinical outcome. In this chapter, malnutrition does not refer to excessive nutrition that is linked to conditions such as obesity.

Risk of malnutrition should be assessed using assessment tools such as the Malnutrition Universal Screening Tool (adult) or the Paediatric Yorkhill Malnutrition Score on admission.

The Nursing Associate determines normal eating habits as part of the admission process (see Box 33.1). Information must be documented within the patient's nutritional care plan. Observe for signs that may indicate that there could be dysphagia (see Box 33.2). Identify those who require support with nutrition; this can include ensuring everything is close to hand and within easy reach and opening packaging or identifying those who need additional assistance by using the red tray or tableware initiative. Where appropriate always seek specialist advice from other colleagues.

Hydration

Often, people who are unwell will not drink enough, and it is important that the Nursing Associate regularly monitors for signs of dehydration (see Box 33.3). Monitoring hydration requires the Nursing Associate to observe, measure and communicate (see Box 33.4). Dehydration that is not monitored and managed can have physiological implications (see Box 33.5). When encouraging hydration, it is essential to ensure that individual preference is taken into account just as individual clinical needs are (see Box 33.6).

Bladder and bowel health

People of all ages can have a problem controlling the bladder or bowel; however, this may become more of a problem as a person gets older and can influence physical, social and psychological health and independence. It is not always easy to talk about bladder and bowel problems, but the Nursing Associate, through a respectful approach, can make this easier.

Understanding and using various approaches and methods of observation, monitoring and recording of a person's bladder and bowel health enables Nursing Associates to provide person-centred, safe and effective care. Promotion of dignity, comfort and privacy are of key importance in this sensitive and intimate area of care.

There are different types and causes of incontinence. Understanding why a person may have bowel and bladder problems with continence determines what the problem is and what treatment is required. Details include the individual's signs and symptoms; a physical examination may be indicated. It is important to identify why the person is seeking advice at this time (see Box 33.7).

The fluid balance chart is a calculation of a person's fluid intake and fluid output. The main objective is to ensure the safe assessment and management of those at risk of fluid balance abnormalities, ensure that fluid balance monitoring is completed consistently and any abnormalities identified are responded to in a timely manner. Fluid balance charts (style and form) vary and usually include an area for documentation of special instructions, consideration of insensible loss and for 24-hour review of fluid balance. There are opportunities for patient involvement in maintaining fluid balance, the Nursing Associate must adhere to local policy and procedure, reporting and recording concerns promptly.

34 Mobility

At the point of registration, the Nursing Associate will be able to: demonstrate the knowledge, skills and ability to act as required to meet people's needs related to mobility, hygiene, oral care, wound care and skin integrity.

Table 34.1 Some disease processes directly affecting mobility.

Nervous system	Musculoskeletal system
• Cerebral palsy • Multiple sclerosis • Parkinson disease	• Muscular dystrophy • Osteoarthritis • Rheumatoid arthritis

Table 34.2 Some hazards of immobility (Source: Adapted Peate and Wild, 2018; Giddens, 2017).

Body system	Impact	Potential complications
Cardiovascular	Blood pooling in extremities Decreased cardiac output	Postural (orthostatic) hypotension Formation of thrombus
Respiratory	Reduced lung expansion Hypoventilation Impaired gaseous exchange Decreased cough reflex Pooling of pulmonary secretions Decrease in respiratory muscle strength	Pneumonia Hypoxaemia Atelectasis (lung collapse) Pulmonary oedema Formation of thrombus Retention of pulmonary secretion
Skin	Oxygen and nutrient delivery to skin decreased Pressure between bed/chair and bony prominences causing tissue ischaemia Skin redness over bony prominences Friction and shearing of skin when moved	Breakdown of skin Excoriation Impaired wound healing Pressure ulcer formation Infection
Gastrointestinal	Reduced peristalsis Anorexia Decreased fluid intake Dysphasia	Malnutrition Constipation Faecal impaction Abdominal distension Flatulence/ileus Nausea/vomiting/indigestion Aspiration Poor oral hygiene
Musculoskeletal	Reduction in muscle mass Muscle strength reduced Impaired joint mobility (shortening and tightening of connective tissue) Compromised calcium metabolism	Tiredness (fatigue) Risk of falls (decreased stability and balance) Muscle atrophy Contractures Osteoporosis Pathological fracture Foot drop

Top Tip

Nursing care that fails to recognise and respect denies people their humanity.

The Nursing Associate at a Glance, First Edition. Ian Peate.
© 2021 John Wiley & Sons Ltd. Published 2021 by John Wiley & Sons Ltd.

Anyone can develop impaired mobility. People with acute or chronic diseases, traumatic injury or chronic pain are at greater risk of experiencing altered mobility and its associated complications. People who are unconscious, for example, are unable to maintain their normal musculoskeletal movement. They are therefore at higher risk of contractures, due to decreased movement and an inability to maintain skin integrity (including wound care) and their hygiene needs (including oral care). The Nursing Associate needs to have the knowledge, skills and capability to intervene as required to meet their needs. Physical mobility requires muscle strength and energy, along with sufficient skeletal stability, joint function and neuromuscular integration. If anything interrupts this process, impaired mobility or immobility could result.

Disease processes

Some disease processes directly affecting mobility are shown in Table 34.1. Other disorders that may impair mobility include congenital deformities, osteochondrodysplasia, diseases contributing to fatigue such as heart failure and chronic obstructive pulmonary disease. Traumatic orthopaedic, head and spinal injuries are likely to impair mobility.

Chronic pain related to various medical disorders and surgical procedures can have an effect on a person's ability to move. Malnutrition and nutritional deficiencies complicate or delay healing and recovery, prolonging immobility impairments.

Injuries associated with falls can also affect mobility. Musculoskeletal and other changes related to ageing, for example, decreased bone density, decreased muscle mass, loss of peripheral vision and dementia can come together to make older adults more prone to falls as well as traumatic injury.

Impaired mobility has negative outcomes for nearly all body systems. If prolonged, immobility leads to deconditioning and loss of function. It has a negative impact on a person's well-being.

The psychosocial effects of immobility are expressed in changes in mood and affect. Those with impaired mobility can become bored and experience anxiety, grief, anger and altered verbal/nonverbal communication responses. Change in mobility status can also alter the person's body image, which can lead to decreased self-esteem and a feeling of powerlessness. The person can withdraw from social interaction, further exacerbating the impact of isolation. Some of the hazards associated with immobility are highlighted in Table 34.2.

Respect

Patients may lose their independence when they access care, putting their dignity at risk. Person-centred care enables the Nursing Associate to maintain that dignity by respecting people's wishes and treating them with compassion and empathy.

Respecting people as individuals is an integral part of all care and is particularly important in the provision of personal hygiene, helping people to go to the toilet and when performing intimate procedures. Respect must underpin the relationship between those who receive care and support and those who are delivering it.

Nursing interventions

Once an assessment of needs has been undertaken, the nursing interventions will depend on the patient's underlying cause(s) of their immobility.

Where possible, immediately addressing mobility needs, acting quickly and safely can be beneficial for the patient's health and well-being, helping the person to achieve their former level of activity and to avoid potential complications.

To avoid or reduce the complications of immobility, when safe to do so and in accordance with the plan of care and working with the patient, mobilise the individual as soon as possible. Mobilisation efforts will depend on the patient's unique circumstances, for example, illness, disease process, investigations and procedures performed and type of surgery. In meeting the fundamental care needs of people related to mobility, hygiene, oral care, wound care and skin integrity, the importance of the nurse–patient relationship in meeting these complex needs is paramount. The nurse is required to discuss with the patient how to best meet their hygiene and personal care needs, for example, by taking into account the individual's level of independence and mobility, interacting with patients in a way that demonstrates compassion and respect, enabling people to be involved in their care and to receive care in a dignified manner. The delivery of such care needs is complex, more than just basic or simple.

35 The deteriorating patient

At the point of registration, the Nursing Associate will be able to: demonstrate the ability to recognise when a person's condition has improved or deteriorated by undertaking health monitoring. Interpret, promptly respond, share findings, and escalate as needed.

Table 35.1 Aspects of prevention.

Component	Discussion
Careful and accurate monitoring	Staff need to understand the importance of careful and accurate monitoring and what it is they are monitoring, understanding cues and knowing the patient. Accountability and responsibility are paramount.
Timely identification of a problem	Awareness and crucially, an understanding of the measurements, what they mean and how to interpret them and what the patient's holistic condition means – what any deviations may imply. Recognising physiological abnormalities
Appropriate and timely intervention based on the problem	Intervening when appropriate and in a timely manner, understanding policy and procedure and adhering to local standards. Departure from normal practice must be justified
Activation of a team response as needed	The Nursing Associate must first and foremost understand their role and responsibilities in escalating concerns. Understanding and an awareness of teams that can make responses, how to activate this and what is expected from them. Always refer to local policy and procedure

Figure 35.1 A systematic approach to raising issues concerning the deteriorating patient.

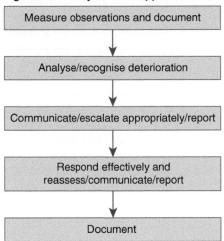

Measure observations and document

↓

Analyse/recognise deterioration

↓

Communicate/escalate appropriately/report

↓

Respond effectively and reassess/communicate/report

↓

Document

Top Tip

Early identification can trigger appropriate management and as such can reduce the need for higher acuity care, reduce hospital lengths of stay and admission costs and in some instances improve survival.

The Nursing Associate at a Glance, First Edition. Ian Peate.
© 2021 John Wiley & Sons Ltd. Published 2021 by John Wiley & Sons Ltd.

Chapter 31 of this text has focused on the need for the Nursing Associate to demonstrate and apply an understanding of how and when they are to escalate to the appropriate professional for expert help and advice with regard to clinical findings. Failure to detect or act to prevent deterioration of the patient whose condition is responsive to treatment is an area of harm that occurs in a number of care settings and is observed in adults and children.

Failing to detect or to act on the deteriorating patient

Failure to rescue is seen as the progressive deterioration in a patient's condition that has not been recognised and prevented, and terminates in death. When healthcare staff fail to detect or to act on the deteriorating patient, treatment may be delayed, which can lead to further patient harm. Failing to detect or to act on the deteriorating patient occurs in a variety of care settings, for example, the inpatient setting, primary care and less acute care settings. Regardless of the setting, such failure adversely impacts the safety of the patient.

Errors in the recognition and management of a deteriorating patient are hardly ever related to a single factor; there is usually a range of multifaceted interactions of system and human factors. When the Nursing Associate understands the complex interaction of systems and those human factors, strategies can be identified that may be used to reduce the possibility of a similar incident occurring. Errors and omissions are seldom related to an intention to do harm.

In order to learn from failures in care, it is important to understand why errors occur. This enables the identification of strategies that may be implemented to reduce the possibility of a similar incident occurring.

Deteriorating patients

Physiological observations are fundamental to the identification of a patient's health status, providing a baseline that enables early identification of clinical deterioration, which makes it possible to improve patient mortality outcomes. In all healthcare environments, the monitoring, measurement, interpretation and prompt response to physiological observations is one of the key roles undertaken by Nursing Associates.

The complications and deterioration associated with failure to rescue (occurring when a generally healthy patient develops complications, deteriorates and as a result subsequently suffers an adverse outcome) are likely involve subtle (and sometimes not so subtle) signs and symptoms that can be dismissed as not being a concern or that are missed entirely. Nursing Associates are key to preventing failure to rescue. There are four aspects of prevention (see Table 35.1). Each of the components in Table 35.1 will require time for direct patient observation. Figure 35.1 details a systematic approach to raising issues concerning the deteriorating patient.

Patients admitted to high dependency or intensive care units are usually connected to systems that provide almost continuous monitoring of multiple variables. In contrast, for patients admitted to the hospital ward, monitoring is often limited to intermittent observations and measurements of a series of physiological parameters, for example, heart rate, respiratory rate and temperature. Yet such patients, often classified as low acuity, can be at risk of sudden, unexpected deterioration.

Factors impeding deterioration

There are a number of factors that can impede recognition of patient deterioration and therefore delayed appropriate and timely escalation of care.

Patient assessment, recording and documentation of vital signs need to be understood as important and not seen as a technical, ritualistic act or 'doing the obs' delegated to the most junior of staff. There is a need consider the value of holistic patient assessment, knowing the patient so as to recognise subtle changes in condition using objective (technical skills) and subjective (non-technical skills) data. Failure to document and report the findings of assessment and when appropriate initiating escalation protocols are further factors. See Chapter 31 for a discussion on the use of SBAR (Situation, Background, Assessment, Recommendation) when calling for help.

When nurses do not seek appropriate support or do not activate a team response, appropriate clinical management and escalation of care can be delayed, thus jeopardising patient safety. Escalating concerns must conform with local policy and procedure.

The value of the Nursing Associates' skills in recognising and responding to patient's deterioration, reducing adverse events and enhancing patient safety should never be understated. The recognition and management of the deteriorating patient is complex and multidimensional. Patient acuity continues to increase as the population becomes older with more complex care needs.

36 Anxiety and confusion

At the point of registration, the Nursing Associate will be able to: Demonstrate the knowledge and skills required to support people with commonly encountered symptoms including anxiety, confusion, discomfort and pain.

Box 36.1 Physical and psychological symptoms of generalised anxiety disorder (GAD) in adults.

- Dizziness
- Fatigue
- Palpitations: fast or irregular heartbeat
- Muscle aches and tension
- Trembling or shaking
- Dry mouth
- Excessive sweating
- Shortness of breath
- Chest pain
- Abdominal pain
- Nausea
- Headache
- Insomnia
- Paraesthesia (pins and needles)
- Restlessness
- A sense of dread
- Feeling constantly 'on edge'
- Depersonalisation
- Difficulty concentrating
- Irritability, exaggerated response to minor surprises or to being startled.

Table 36.1 The Stepped Care Model (NICE, 2019).

Step	Intervention
1: All known and suspected presentations of GAD	Identification, assessment, education, monitoring
2: Diagnosed GAD that has not improved after education and active monitoring in primary care	Low-intensity psychological support, non-facilitated or guided self-help, psycho-educational groups
3: GAD with an inadequate response to step 2 interventions or marked functional impairment	Cognitive behavioural therapy (CBT)/applied relaxation or drug treatment
4: Complex treatment – refractory GAD and very marked functional impairment, such as self-neglect or a high risk of self-harm	Specialist drug and/or psychological treatment, multi-agency teams, crisis intervention, outpatient or inpatient care

Box 36.2 Risk factors associated with an increased risk of delirium.

- Those over 65 years
- Male
- Pre-existing cognitive deficit – dementia, stroke
- Severity of dementia
- Severe comorbidity
- Previous episode of delirium
- Some types of operation – hip fracture repairs, emergency operations
- Certain conditions - burns, fractures, infection, low albumin, dehydration
- Severe illness
- Drug use and dependence – e.g. benzodiazepines
- Substance misuse – e.g. alcohol
- Extremes of sensory experience – e.g. hypothermia or hyperthermia
- Visual or hearing problems
- Poor mobility
- Social isolation
- Stress
- Terminally ill
- Movement to a new environment
- Intensive care unit admission
- Urea/creatinine abnormalities

Top Tip
Sudden confusion (delirium) can have many different causes. Seek medical help immediately if someone suddenly becomes confused (delirious).

The Nursing Associate at a Glance, First Edition. Ian Peate.
© 2021 John Wiley & Sons Ltd. Published 2021 by John Wiley & Sons Ltd.

This chapter discusses the knowledge and skills required to support people with commonly encountered symptoms including anxiety and confusion. Discomfort and pain are discussed in Chapter 37.

Generalised anxiety disorder

Generalised anxiety disorder (GAD) is a syndrome of ongoing anxiety and worry about many events or thoughts that a patient generally recognises as excessive and inappropriate. The condition can be chronic and debilitating. The severity of the symptoms will vary from person to person. Some people may only have one or two symptoms, others have many more.

Prevalence and risk

Prevalence is difficult to determine. Numbers are higher for women than for men. There are different rates across cultural groups, and the condition is more prevalent in elderly populations. Risk factors include age between 35 and 54 years, being divorced or separated, living alone or as a lone parent. Protective factors have been identified, including age between 16 and 24 years, being married or cohabiting.

Symptoms

There are a number of physical symptoms of GAD (see Box 36.1). Symptoms can cause the person to withdraw from social contact to avoid feelings of worry and dread. They may also find going to work difficult and stressful and may take time off sick. These actions can increase anxiety even more and intensify lack of self-esteem.

Treatment and support

Nursing interventions must be person centred and recovery based to ensure accurate diagnosis, implementation of appropriate person-centred treatment and enable best level of functioning and quality of life. The Nursing Associate works collaboratively with the patient, providing support, education and appropriate treatment to enhance patient outcomes and quality of life.

The stepped-care model for treatment of GAD suggests offering the least intrusive, most effective intervention first. The initial steps concentrate on identification and assessment, followed by low-intensity interventions and more complex specialist treatments if required (see Table 36.1). Psychological therapies (such as cognitive behavioural therapy (CBT)) and pharmacological therapies are based on the age of the patient, previous treatment response, risks of deliberate self-harm or accidental overdose, tolerability, possible interactions with existing medications and patient's preference.

Confusion

Acute confusion, sometimes called acute confessional state or delirium, is an acute cognitive impairment accompanied by a severe illness. The condition can fluctuate going through cycles of improving and then worsening. Delirium can be hypoactive or hyperactive, but some people show signs of both (mixed). Risk factors are shown in Box 36.2.

Symptoms

Common symptoms in patients with hyperactive delirium include disturbances in sleep and concentration, agitation, heightened arousal, aggression and restlessness. These patients may also experience hallucinations and extremes of mood. Patients with hypoactive delirium are often quiet, sleepy, withdrawn, lethargic and apathetic, and have reduced alertness and slurred speech. Certain medications can cause acute confusion.

Treatment and support

Nursing Associates need to understand the risk factors for delirium and be aware of the symptoms, addressing risk factors where possible. When acute confusion has been acknowledged, vital signs and hydration status are assessed as well as any potentially reversible causes of the confusion to identify the specific cause. A delay in treatment may result in poorer patient outcomes.

The care environment can exacerbate acute confusion. Therefore, changing environments by moving a patient should be avoided unless this is absolutely necessary. Minimise excessive noise; this can reduce agitation. If there are any language deficits (as result of central nervous infection, for example), consider using simplified communication, for example, simple, direct words for objects and commands, and pictures and letter boards to help patients communicate. Patients may become verbally and physically aggressive when they are acutely confused. Use de-escalation techniques. If a person with delirium is distressed or considered a risk to themselves or others, de-escalation techniques are ineffective. Consider giving short-term (usually for 1 week or less) haloperidol. Start at the lowest clinically appropriate dose, and titrate cautiously according to symptoms. Antipsychotic drugs should be used with caution.

37 Discomfort and pain

At the point of registration, the Nursing Associate will be able to: demonstrate the knowledge and skills required to support people with commonly encountered symptoms including anxiety, confusion, discomfort and pain.

Box 37.1   Possible signs of pain.

- Becoming restless or trying to hold or rub a particular part of the body
- Grimacing or making moaning sounds
- Becoming agitated, irritable or aggressive
- Sweating, cool clammy skin, tachycardia, tachypnoea, hypertension
- Being unable to rest or sleep
- Withdrawal

Table 37.1 Some common misconceptions about the nature of pain (McGann, 2007).

You can teach people to tolerate pain; the longer they have it, the more used to it they will become.	False. Tolerance to pain is an individual experience. People with prolonged pain tend to develop pain hypersensitivity.
Nursing staff and other clinicians are the authority on pain and the nature of pain.	False. The patient experiencing the pain fully understands how it feels and its impact on their life.
Lying about the existence of pain or shirking is common.	Very few people lie about the existence of pain, and being dishonest about pain is rare.
Visible symptoms of pain can be used to prove its severity.	Not always – lack of pain expression does not imply lack of pain. Those living with chronic pain may have the ability to carry on as normal.
Patients should not be given analgesia until a reason for their pain has been diagnosed.	This would not ensure holistic or person-centred care. Pain should be treated even when there is no apparent cause. People seeking assistance for pain have the right to have their pain assessed, accepted and acted upon.

Box 37.2   Pain classification.

- Transient pain – A short episode of pain, occurring as a result of a minor injury. This pain can be intense, causing upset. However, it will be short-lived and temporary. In most cases, the individual will consider the pain to be unimportant and not seek medical attention.
- Acute pain – Debilitating pain, has a sudden onset and continues until healing begins. The pain experience will be prolonged and continue until healing begins. Individuals in acute pain may describe it as intolerable and intense.
- Chronic pain – Pain that continues even though healing is complete. The pain becomes a permanent feature of an individual's life and can have a lasting effect on the person's well-being.

Top Tip

Promoting comfort and easing suffering and pain are fundamental elements of nursing practice.

The Nursing Associate at a Glance, First Edition. Ian Peate.
© 2021 John Wiley & Sons Ltd. Published 2021 by John Wiley & Sons Ltd.

This chapter discusses the knowledge and skills required to support people in pain and to promote comfort. Confusion and anxiety are discussed in Chapter 36.

Pain

Pain is the most likely reason people seek medical assistance. Everyone experiences pain periodically, throughout their life, although it is difficult to define. It is unpleasant and an uncomfortable sensation, occurring as a result of injury, inflammation or disease. Pain can also be constant in those with a long-term health condition (physical pain is termed nociceptive). Pain is also a term used to describe our emotional state, our feelings. Pain is a unique and personal experience, and the way in which someone expresses and deals with their pain will depend on their culture, life experiences and personality. Pain is what the person says it is, and the intensity of pain sensation depends on what pain means to the individual (see Box 37.1).

People's needs when in pain and also at the end of their life will vary. There will be physical needs for food and fluids, personal hygiene and the need for comfort and psychological needs as the person in pain may be frightened. There will be social needs, with the person anxious about family and work issues. Spiritual needs can also be apparent with the person seeking either religious or non-religious spiritual comfort.

Pain can cause great distress for the patient and those around them. The team offering care and support listen to the patient and assess the best approach to pain management. This may be a combination of medications and non-pharmaceutical approaches with the aim of keeping the person as comfortable as possible. The Nursing Associate offers support by reporting rapidly any signs that the patient is in pain. Some of the signs to observe for are highlighted in Box 37.1. There are many misconceptions concerning what pain is and the best way to treat it. Many of the beliefs about pain and pain relief are false (see Table 37.1).

Acute and chronic pain management

Acute pain is defined as pain that occurs for less than three months; chronic pain is often defined as that which persists beyond three to six months (see Box 37.2).

A key element of nursing care is the effective management of acute and chronic pain. The Nursing Associate is with the patient for extended periods of time providing direct patient care, so they are well placed to monitor and manage acute and chronic pain. The Nursing Associate has the important responsibility of ensuring the safe use of analgesics and to carry out regular reviews of the effectiveness of these medicines as well as any non-pharmaceutical interventions. The Nursing Associate can educate patients on the use of non- pharmacological self-management strategies and by making appropriate referrals to pain management resources. However, doing this safely and effectively requires a comprehensive knowledge of pain management strategies and guidance, updating knowledge and accessing up-to-date evidence on pain management.

A structured approach

Structured pain assessment has to be performed as part of effective pain management. The Nursing Associate needs to understand how they can improve the provision of analgesics and the patients' ability to perform the activities of living.

In chronic pain management, the focus should be on non-pharmacological strategies as much as on the use of analgesic drugs. Prescription medication for chronic pain is the most convenient aspect of care. However, it is potentially the most harmful and sometimes the least effective. Psychological elements are an essential component of the pain experience. Non-pharmacological methods of pain management can ease anxiety or stress, helping the person to manage their pain. The most effective, evidence-based, psychological treatment for chronic pain is cognitive behavioural therapy, involving a series of structured, patient-focussed sessions aiming to address the person's psychological and emotional experience of their pain.

Listening to the patient and tailoring care to their needs demonstrates you are proficient in providing and evaluating care for the individual living with pain. Acknowledge what is important to people and use this insight to ensure that their needs for safety, dignity, privacy, comfort and sleep can be met. Act as a role model for others as you provide evidence-based person-centred care.

Nursing Associates should never assume that a patient cannot participate in a pain assessment. Self-report pain scales can be used, but people need to be taught how to use them. Patients change their 'usual' behaviour when they are in pain; therefore, knowing individual patients and their normal behaviours is vital.

38 End-of-life care

At the point of registration, the Nursing Associate will be able to: demonstrate an understanding of how to deliver sensitive and compassionate end-of-life care to support people to plan for their end of life, giving information and support to people who are dying, their families and the bereaved. Provide care to the deceased.

Figure 38.1   Various steps associated with end-of-life care (NHS, 2014).

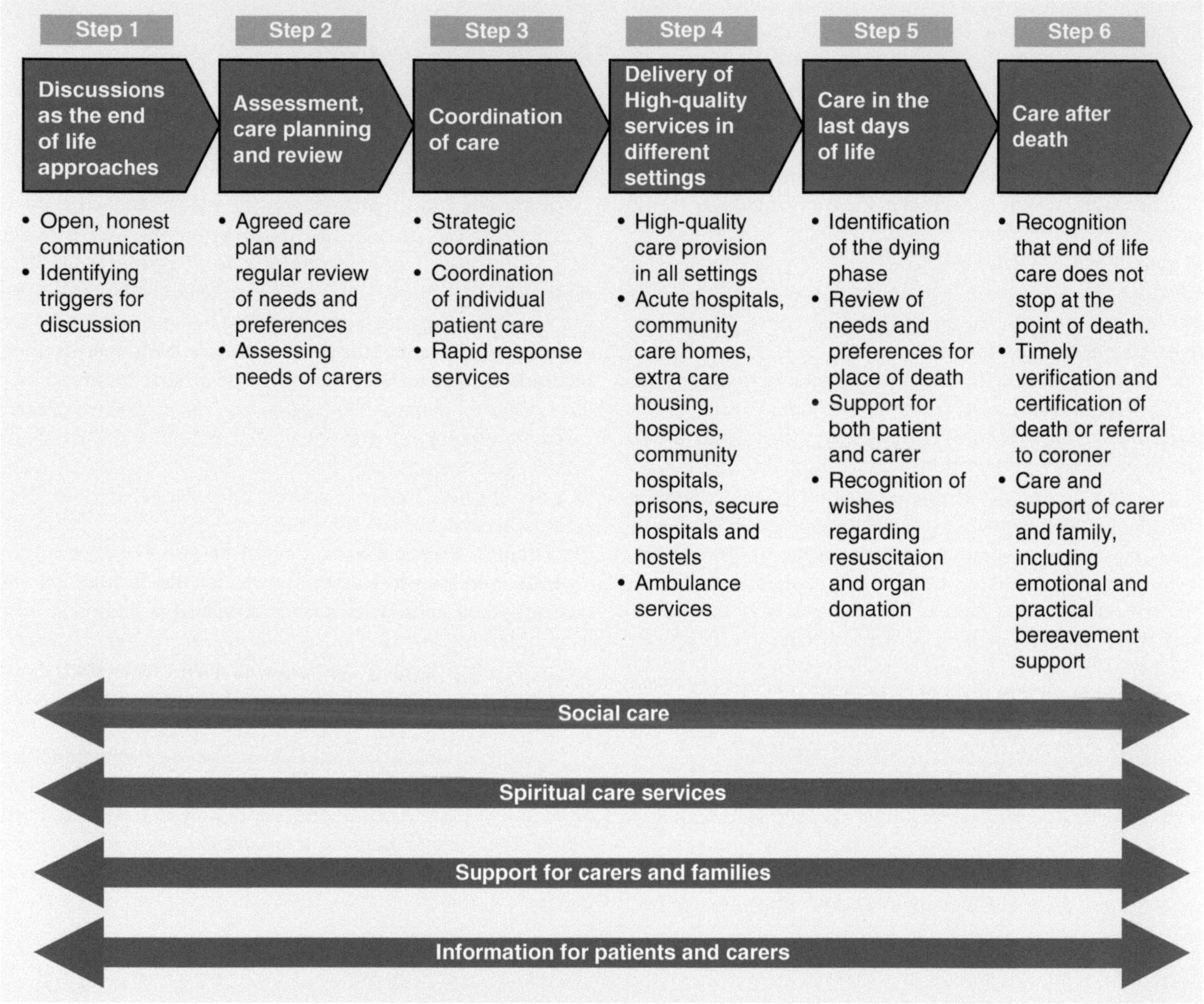

Step 1	Step 2	Step 3	Step 4	Step 5	Step 6
Discussions as the end of life approaches	**Assessment, care planning and review**	**Coordination of care**	**Delivery of High-quality services in different settings**	**Care in the last days of life**	**Care after death**
• Open, honest communication • Identifying triggers for discussion	• Agreed care plan and regular review of needs and preferences • Assessing needs of carers	• Strategic coordination • Coordination of individual patient care • Rapid response services	• High-quality care provision in all settings • Acute hospitals, community care homes, extra care housing, hospices, community hospitals, prisons, secure hospitals and hostels • Ambulance services	• Identification of the dying phase • Review of needs and preferences for place of death • Support for both patient and carer • Recognition of wishes regarding resuscitaion and organ donation	• Recognition that end of life care does not stop at the point of death. • Timely verification and certification of death or referral to coroner • Care and support of carer and family, including emotional and practical bereavement support

← Social care →

← Spiritual care services →

← Support for carers and families →

← Information for patients and carers →

Top Tip

How we care for the dying is a sign of how we care for all people who are sick and for those who are vulnerable; it is a measure of society as a whole.

The Nursing Associate at a Glance, First Edition. Ian Peate.
© 2021 John Wiley & Sons Ltd. Published 2021 by John Wiley & Sons Ltd.

At the end of life, everyone has the right to be cared for with dignity and respect.

End of life

The term *end of life* is often referred to as the last year of life, but for some people this will be significantly shorter. End of life and the term *palliative care* are sometimes used interchangeably. Palliative care largely relates to symptom management, rather than to actual end-of-life care. End-of-life care is the responsibility of the Nursing Associate and all nurses, not only specialist nurses and teams. This kind of care should be made available in all settings, working with the patient and if appropriate their family also.

End-of-life care does not focus solely on the practical and technical aspects of care delivery. It also refers to the support and information available to the patient and those people who are important to them, as well encompassing bereavement support.

Ethics

Patients who are dying are entitled to receive the same standard of care as all other patients. To be treated with dignity and respect throughout, privacy and dignity must be respected, and good-quality care provided in comfortable surroundings. Patients and those close to them must be treated with understanding and compassion.

The Nursing Associate offers support to those who are approaching the end of their lives, in a sensitive and compassionate way, maintaining nutrition and hydration that reflects individual needs and preference. These elements of care are very often complex, and they involve ethical considerations. Any decision made must be based on a holistic assessment of needs with the patient leading this and supported by an experienced senior clinician. Figure 38.1 considers the various steps that associated with end-of-life care. Chapter 39 of this text discusses end-of-life decisions and orders.

Recognising end of life

Recognising the factors that may indicate that a person is in the last days or hours of life is complex and subtle, and the Nursing Associate needs to be aware of the psychological effects of the dying phase/last days of life for an individual and the key theories and models relating to loss and grief. For some, death is slower and gradual, and for others, death can come suddenly. In some, the body fails whereas the mind stays alert; and others remain physically strong, but their mind declines.

As a person approaches the end of life, they may sleep more, and they can be difficult to wake at times. There may be loss of appetite and confusion, and the person may not remember familiar faces. Restlessness can occur, and the person might pull at bedclothes and have visions of people or things that are not really there. They may develop a fixed stare. Bladder and bowel control may be lost. Secretions can collect at the back of the throat, and this can sound like a rattle. As the circulation slows down, the person's legs and arms can feel pale and appear purple, bluish and mottled. The face becomes pale, and breathing becomes irregular and can stop for short periods. The pulse becomes fast and irregular.

It is normally possible and desirable to meet the wishes of a dying person. However, when this is not possible, explain the reason to the person who is dying and those important to them. The dying process can be stressful for those around the patient, and support will be needed to help relatives and loved ones as death approaches. Offer gentle, and if needed, repeated explanations regarding the care that is being given; the ineffectiveness of any treatment, nutrition and hydration attempts; and the fact that these events are irreversible. During those final minutes, explain to people that touch is also a form of communication, and encourage everyone to say their goodbyes.

When death has occurred

Depending on the circumstances, once death has occurred, the provision of care needs to be focused on those in the room. Allow people to spend time with the body, within the cultural and clinical limits allowed. This can give them an opportunity to make sense of what has happened.

Even after a person has died, the Nursing Associate must continue to provide individualised care, respecting personal wishes, spiritual, cultural and religious beliefs. Caring for a person after death (sometimes known as last offices) is the final act that the Nursing Associate will carry out for the patient. The Nursing Associate should always seek advice and support for this final act of caring, ensuring the patient's personal wishes have been respected and local policy and procedure have been adhered to.

39 End-of-life decisions and orders

At the point of registration, the Nursing Associate will be able to: understand and act in line with any end-of-life decisions and orders, organ and tissue donation protocols, infection protocols, advanced planning decisions, living wills and lasting powers of attorney for health.

Table 39.1 Having end-of-life conversations.

When to have end-of-life conversations
• When the person has an advanced progressing life-limiting illness (for example, cancer, heart disease, chronic obstructive pulmonary disease)
• A prognosis of 6–12 months
• The person has a treatment decision to make
• When referred to palliative care
• Patient's treatment is not working

How to have end-of-life conversations
• Make eye contact
• Sit close to the person
• Provide time and silence
• Listen, reflect and respect
• Demonstrate compassion
• Initiate conversation about concerns regarding the future and dying
• Avoid medical jargon
• Offer emotional support

What to discuss
• Outline what advanced care planning is about and power of attorney
• Discuss DNAR and what this means (code status)
• If appropriate, introduce hypothetical situations
• With whom and how you will share the information given

Top Tip

Those who are approaching the end of their life require high-quality care, supporting them to live as well as possible until they die, and to die with dignity.

The Nursing Associate at a Glance, First Edition. Ian Peate.
© 2021 John Wiley & Sons Ltd. Published 2021 by John Wiley & Sons Ltd.

The law

End-of-life decisions and orders must take account of, and be consistent with, current law across the UK, including the laws on decision-making for patients who lack capacity, the law that prohibits killing (including euthanasia) and assisting suicide, and the requirements of the Human Rights Act 1998. The Nursing Associate must always seek advice if there is uncertainty about issues associated with end-of-life decisions and orders.

Approaching the end of life

Patients can be said to be 'approaching the end of life' when they are likely to die within the next 12 months. This includes patients whose death is imminent (expected within a few hours or days) and those with:

- Advanced, progressive, incurable conditions
- General frailty and co-existing conditions that mean they are expected to die within 12 months
- Existing conditions if they are at risk of dying from a sudden acute crisis in their condition
- Life-threatening acute conditions caused by sudden catastrophic events.

Advance care planning

As the person approaches the dying phase (see Chapter 38), the multi-professional team undertakes a review of the patient's treatment plan and medication. It may be necessary to complete a Do Not Attempt Resuscitation (DNAR) order if not already established. This will be undertaken by the GP responsible for the patient at home or in a care home; the medical team will complete this in the hospital or hospice. Wherever possible, the patient should be included in this decision unless to do so would cause the patient extreme distress. An advance directive may be in place, aiding decision making.

The generic term *advance care planning* is used to describe a structured discussion about a person's wishes and thoughts concerning their care at the end of life. Some patients will decide to document what their wishes are in a formal way, years in advance, whereas others may have discussions once a palliative diagnosis had been made, or they are told they are approaching the end of their life. Advance care planning is often initiated by a member of the specialist palliative care team, or the patient might have had a discussion concerning their wishes with their GP. A copy of an Advance Statement or Lasting Power of Attorney for Health may be present in the patient's records (in the patient's home, hospital, hospice or nursing home).

An advance statement may include commentary in relation to care and treatment, as well as beliefs, cultural wishes and other likes and dislikes. When prepared in advance, this helps the family and carers ensure that wishes are met should the individual lose capacity for decision-making or if they become very sleepy or unconscious as they approach the final stages of life.

The advance decision, sometimes called a living will, is a legally binding document focused on treatment and care wishes which can include whether the patient wishes to be resuscitated, whether they would like to have antibiotics to treat an infection, or if they would want to be admitted to hospital for acute care if their condition suddenly deteriorates. A medical practitioner has to provide a counter signature for an advanced decision – often the patient's GP, unless completed in an acute care environment.

Lasting power of attorney for health and welfare is a legally binding document; the patient passes over the responsibility for decision-making for care and treatment to another. The individual has to have mental capacity when creating a lasting power of attorney, and it must be registered with the Office of the Public Guardian. The lasting power of attorney will only come into effect when a patient no longer has the capacity to make decisions about their own treatment and care.

Discussing death

Discussing the subject of death and a patient's preferences for what they see as a good death can be difficult for a number of reasons, and this becomes even more difficult when there is limited time available. Many Nursing Associates and other healthcare workers can feel uncomfortable asking about end-of-life choices, and they may not feel equipped to handle any questions that arise. However, having such conversations often brings with them positive outcomes, particularly as the discussions may provide the basis for a treatment plan that is more aligned to the patients' preferences for care (see Table 39.1).

40 Medicines management I

At the point of registration, the Nursing Associate will be able to: understand the principles of safe and effective administration and optimisation of medicines in accordance with local and national policies.

Figure 40.1   Principles of medicine optimisation (Source: Adapted Royal Pharmaceutical Society, 2013).

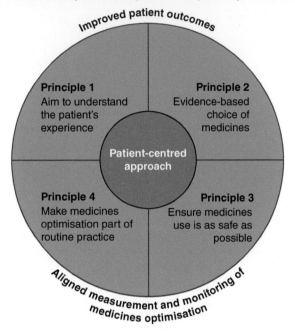

Improved patient outcomes

Principle 1
Aim to understand the patient's experience

Principle 2
Evidence-based choice of medicines

Patient-centred approach

Principle 4
Make medicines optimisation part of routine practice

Principle 3
Ensure medicines use is as safe as possible

Aligned measurement and monitoring of medicines optimisation

Top Tip

The Nursing Associate's role is regulated under statute and aligned with the Code; they must demonstrate the competence required to administer prescribed medicines safely.

The Nursing Associate at a Glance, First Edition. Ian Peate.
© 2021 John Wiley & Sons Ltd. Published 2021 by John Wiley & Sons Ltd.

As more people are taking more medicines, it is becoming increasingly important to get the most from medicines for patients and the NHS. Medicines prevent, treat or manage a number of illnesses or conditions. They are the most common intervention in healthcare. The employer decides whether Nursing Associates administer medicines in their service and the extent of that role.

As part of their role, Nursing Associates may supply, dispense and administer medicines and are educated to understand medicines management and within the confines of local employer policies, administer prescribed medicines safely and appropriately. It is essential that Nursing Associates have been deemed competent in the relevant components of this area so that they can make a full contribution to the provision of effective care to the public and patients in primary, acute, secondary, community and social care settings.

Medicines optimisation

NICE (2015) defined medicines optimisation as 'a person-centred approach to safe and effective medicines use, to ensure people obtain the best possible outcomes from their medicines'. Medicines optimisation is akin to medicines management. The four principles associated with national guidance and good practice guidance supports medicines optimisation and are depicted in Figure 40.1.

Principle 1 – understanding the patent's experience

To ensure the best possible outcomes from medicines use, there must be ongoing, open dialogue with the patient and/or their carer about the patient's choice, acknowledging and taking into account their experience of using medicines to manage their condition; noting that the patient's experience can change over time even if the medicines do not. Understanding the patient's experience demonstrates recognition and acceptance of the need for patient-centred care approaches in the delivery of services.

Principle 2 – choice of medicines

In ensuring that the needs of the patient are paramount, the most appropriate choice of clinically and cost-effective medicines should be made available. This choice has to be informed by the best available evidence.

Principle 3 – safe use of medicines

The safe use of medicines is the responsibility of all health and social care professionals, health and care organisations and patients. Safe use should be discussed with patients and/or their carers. Safety concerns medicines usage, including unwanted effects, interactions, processes and systems and effective communication between professionals.

Patient safety incidents can be related to errors in the process of prescribing, preparing, dispensing, administering, monitoring and providing advice on medicines.

Principle 4 – medicines optimisation as part of routine practice

The Nursing Associate and other health and care professionals should, as a matter of routine, discuss with each other and with patients and/or their carers how to maximise outcomes from medicines.

Regular review of a patient's medication is an example, ensuring that medicines optimisation becomes part of routine practice. This is a structured, critical examination of a person's medicines, working with them and reaching an agreement about treatment, optimising the impact of medicines, reducing the number of medication-related problems as well as reducing waste.

Effective administration of medicines

The Nursing Associate is required to follow a number of local and national policies so as to administer medicines safely. By being familiar with the medications that are to be administered, adhering to policy and implementing safeguards, you can help protect patients from harm and ensure their medicine are having the desired effects.

There are several ways of ensuring that medicines are administered safely; these are the nine rights of medication administration:

1 Right patient
2 Right medication
3 Right route
4 Right dose
5 Right time
6 Right documentation
7 Right action
8 Right form
9 Right response.

41 Medicines management II

At the point of registration, the Nursing Associate will be able to: demonstrate the ability to recognise the effects of medicines, allergies, drug sensitivity, side effects, contraindications and adverse reactions.

Box 41.1 Anaphylaxis.

If a medication is administered after a 'sensitising dose', this second exposure or dose has the potential to lead to anaphylaxis, or anaphylactic shock. The signs and symptoms of anaphylaxis and anaphylactic shock are:

- Decreased cardiac output
- Drop in blood pressure
- Tachycardia with a bounding pulse
- Laryngeal oedema
- Respiratory distress

    Unless anaphylaxis is treated immediately, it can lead to death.

Table 41.1 Type A and B adverse drug reactions.

Type A	Type B
Common and predictable and associated with the pharmacological actions of a drug.	Not associated with the known pharmacology of a drug. Type B reactions are rare, but when they occur they can result in severe illness and death.

Top Tip

The prime goal of nursing care is to maximise health and well-being and in so doing to optimise the quality of people's lives.

The Nursing Associate at a Glance, First Edition. Ian Peate.
© 2021 John Wiley & Sons Ltd. Published 2021 by John Wiley & Sons Ltd.

Medicines are the most common intervention in healthcare. They have a crucial role in preventing illness, managing long-term conditions and curing disease. Some medicines can cause an adverse reaction in the patient, or an adverse effect may occur. Any drug may produce unwanted or unexpected adverse reactions. Rapid detection and recording of adverse drug reactions is of vital importance so that unrecognised hazards are identified quickly and appropriate action is taken to ensure that medicines are used safely.

The effects of medicines

The administration of medicines involves much more than handing the prescribed medicine to a patient. The administration of medication entails the Nursing Associate's application of critical thinking skills, the use of professional judgement, their application of pathophysiology, a detailed understanding of the patient and their condition and the effects of the medicines

When medicines are prescribed, the Nursing Associate must be knowledgeable about the indications, contraindications, side effects, adverse effects as well as the interactions associated with the medication. A reliable resource would be the British National Formulary (BNF) and British National Formulary Child (BNFc).

If the Nursing Associate has any concerns about any prescription, it must be questioned and the prescriber contacted so that a discussion about those concerns can begin. Once the medicine has been administered, the Nursing Associate is responsible and accountable for closely monitoring the patient for any side effects and adverse actions.

Contraindications

Nearly all medications have contraindications against their use. A contraindication is a specific situation in which a drug should not be used as it may be harmful to the person. Some of the most commonly occurring contraindications for medications include:

- Sensitivity or allergy to the medication
- Pregnancy
- Breast feeding
- Renal disease
- Hepatic disease

Prior to the administration of medicines, the Nursing Associate must be fully knowledgeable about the contraindications of the medications, the person's condition and be able to determine whether or not the prescribed medication is contraindicated for the patient. When the Nursing Associate identifies that a medication is contraindicated for a patient, they must communicate with the prescriber so as to clarify the prescription.

Allergy and drug sensitivity

Allergic reactions to medications may be minor, but they can also be very serious and life threatening. Therefore, the Nursing Associate must assess the patient and identify any potential allergies.

All allergies are documented and reported according to local policy (for example, in the nursing assessment and also on the prescription). Allergy bands and/or bar codes may be used with embedded allergy information, enabling staff to readily identify allergies to medications.

First exposure to penicillin, for example, is referred to as the 'sensitising dose', sensitising and preparing the body to respond to a second exposure or dose. The signs and symptoms of this allergic 'sensitising dose' response can include a body-wide rash and itching. When this is observed, discontinue the medication, notify the prescriber and doctor, and document this reaction according to local policy. See Box 41.1 for a discussion concerning anaphylaxis.

Adverse drug reaction

An adverse drug reaction (ADR) is a harmful or unwanted reaction experienced after a drug or combination of drugs has been administered under normal conditions of use, related to or is suspected to be related to the drug. There are two types of ADR (see Table 41.1). Reporting of ADRs in the UK is undertaken via the Yellow Card Scheme. Yellow cards are available in the BNF, or online at the Medicines and Healthcare products Regulatory Agency (MHRA) website (https://www.gov.uk/report-problem-medicine-medical-device).

The scheme helps the MHRA to identify previously unrecognised or suspected ADRs, and provides valuable information on recognised adverse drug reactions.

Some patients may confuse a side effect with an allergic reaction. Side effects, for example, nausea, diarrhoea and sedation, are often reported as allergies, when in fact no immunological mechanism is involved. The Nursing Associate needs to inform the patient of any potential side effects.

42 Medicines management III

At the point of registration, the Nursing Associate will be able to: recognise the different ways by which medicines can be prescribed.

Table 42.1 Some routes of administration.

Route	
Oral	By mouth
Injection	Intravenously, intramuscularly, intrathecally, subcutaneously, intradermally
Implantation	Under the skin
Sublingual	Under the tongue
Buccal	Between the gums and cheek
Ocular	In the eye
Otic	In the ear
Nasal	Into the nose
Inhalation	Into the lungs
Topical	Having effect at the site of application
Transdermal	Through the skin
Pessary	In to the vagina
Suppository	In to the rectum

Figure 42.1 Drug administration.

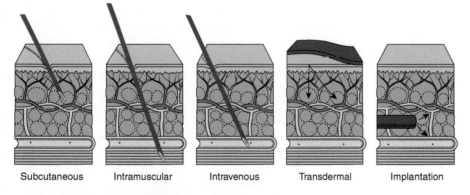

Subcutaneous   Intramuscular   Intravenous   Transdermal   Implantation

Figure 42.2 Sublingual and buccal routes.

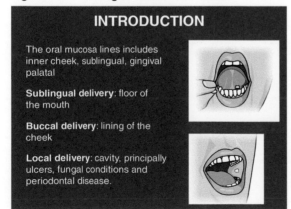

INTRODUCTION

The oral mucosa lines includes inner cheek, sublingual, gingival palatal

Sublingual delivery: floor of the mouth

Buccal delivery: lining of the cheek

Local delivery: cavity, principally ulcers, fungal conditions and periodontal disease.

Top Tip

The route through which a drug is administered is important. The Nursing Associates must always give this consideration, always acting the best interests of the patient.

The Nursing Associate at a Glance, First Edition. Ian Peate.
© 2021 John Wiley & Sons Ltd. Published 2021 by John Wiley & Sons Ltd.

Most medicines come in a variety of types or formulations. Medicines can be introduced into the body in different ways, and the prescription reflects this. See Table 42.1 and Figure 42.1 for the various routes of administration.

Oral

Many drugs can be administered orally as liquids, capsules, tablets or chewable tablets. The oral route is used most often and is the most convenient; usually it is the safest and least expensive route. It can have limitations because of how a drug usually moves through the gastrointestinal tract. Absorption may begin in the mouth and stomach, and most drugs are usually absorbed from the small intestine. The drug passes through the intestinal wall, travelling to the liver prior to being transported via the bloodstream to the target site. The intestinal wall and liver chemically metabolise many drugs, thus decreasing the amount of drug reaching the bloodstream. Because of this, these drugs are often given in smaller doses when injected intravenously so as to produce the same effect. When administered orally, food and other drugs in the digestive tract can affect how much of and how fast the drug will be absorbed. Some drugs therefore should be taken on an empty stomach, whilst others should be taken with food. Others should not be taken with certain other drugs, and others cannot be administered orally at all. Some orally administered drugs irritate the digestive tract, such as aspirin, and most other non-steroidal anti-inflammatories can damage the lining of the stomach and small intestine. Some other drugs are absorbed poorly or ad hoc in the gastrointestinal tract or are destroyed by the acid and digestive enzymes in the stomach.

Other routes of administration will be needed when the oral route cannot be used, for example, when a person cannot take anything by mouth, when a drug must be administered rapidly or in a precise or very high dose or when a drug is poorly or erratically absorbed from the gastrointestinal tract.

Injection

Parenteral administration is administration by injection (see Table 42.1). The drug can be prepared in ways that prolong drug absorption from the injection site for hours, days or even longer. Such products do not need to be administered as often as drug products with more rapid absorption; a depot injection, for example, is a slow-release, slow-acting form of medication.

Sublingual and buccal

There are some drugs placed sublingually or buccally (see Figure 42.2), permitting them to dissolve and be absorbed directly into the small blood vessels; these drugs are not swallowed. The sublingual route is particularly good for the absorption of glyceryl trinitrate (GTN), used to relieve angina, as absorption is rapid and the drug enters the bloodstream immediately without first passing through the intestinal wall and liver.

Rectal

Most drugs administered orally can also be administered rectally as a suppository. The drug is mixed with a waxy substance, dissolving or liquefying after insertion into the rectum. The wall of the rectum is thin and has a rich blood supply; the drug is readily absorbed. A suppository is prescribed for those who cannot take a drug orally because they have nausea, dysphagia or nil by mouth. Drugs that can be administered rectally include paracetamol (for pyrexia), diazepam (for seizures) and laxatives (for constipation). Drugs that cause irritation in suppository form may need to be administered by injection.

Inhalation and nebulisation

Medication can be provided in droplets so that the drugs can pass through the trachea into the lungs. Smaller droplets will go deeper, increasing the amount of drug absorbed. Inside the lungs, they are absorbed into the bloodstream. Specialised equipment may be needed to administer the drug via this route. Usually, this method is used to administer drugs that act specifically in the lungs, for example, aerosolised antiasthmatic drugs in metered-dose containers (inhalers) and to administer anaesthetic gases used for general anaesthesia.

Nebulisation is similar to the inhalation route. Drugs given by nebulisation have to be aerosolised into small particles to reach the lungs. Nebulisation requires the use of special devices, such as ultrasonic or jet nebuliser systems, helping to maximise the amount of drug delivered to the lungs. Using the device properly helps prevent side effects.

43 Working in partnership with people, families and carers

At the point of registration, the Nursing Associate will be able to: demonstrate the ability to monitor the effectiveness of care in partnership with people, families and carers; document progress and report outcomes.

Figure 43.1 Patient-centred care (Source: Adapted Health Foundation, 2016).

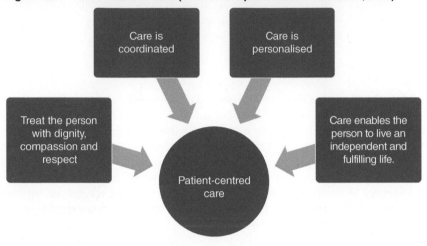

Top Tip
People have a right, in law, to be involved in their care, as set out in the fundamental standard of 'person-centred care', a standard below which care should never fall.

The Nursing Associate at a Glance, First Edition. Ian Peate.
© 2021 John Wiley & Sons Ltd. Published 2021 by John Wiley & Sons Ltd.

The person-centred care approach provides people with more choice and control in their lives by providing a method that is appropriate to the individual's needs. It requires the Nursing Associate and others to change the conversation by asking 'what matters to you' instead of asking 'what is the matter with you', empowering patients, families and carers to take an active role in managing their own health and well-being, and working alongside service providers. The Nursing Associate needs to know what matters to the patient – acknowledging that no two people are the same, listening carefully to the person's views and concerns.

Partnership working

Creating a health and care service where the Nursing Associate no longer does things 'to and for' patients but works with them as equal partners in their own care is central to health strategy, policy and reform. Healthcare services are required to reflect the needs of patients, carers and staff based on their actual experience. It provides a mechanism whereby patients' experiences provide insights which identify opportunities, and they contribute fully to the change process, leading to safer, more dignified, effective and reliable care.

Policies and initiatives have been put in place to increase patient rights so they are able to choose services, help people to take more control over their own health and to support patients. People who use services are becoming more knowledgeable and are demanding a more open and more equitable system of decision-making.

Working in partnership is well established in the NHS Constitution, and NHS staff pledge to work in partnership with patient, families, carers and representatives. The Constitution makes clear that patients will be included in discussions regarding the planning of their care, offered information that they can understand and provided with appropriate support to help them to participate fully in decision-making about healthcare. People often find that they are happier with their care and more likely to adhere to any treatments or care plans when they make decisions jointly with their health or care professional. Partnership working is closely aligned with promoting choice and shared decision-making, whereby healthcare professionals and patients work together to choose investigations, treatment, management and care, all based on the available evidence and the patients' informed preference.

Information provided to patients to help them identify their chosen preferences has to be communicated in ways that are accessible to people with different literacy levels and those with communication difficulties. The Nursing Associate needs to determine service users' preferences and concerns; develop an effective understanding of shared decision-making and empowerment, and be willing and confident to share decision-making equally with them.

Person-centred care

Partnership working and shared decision-making are parallel approaches to person-centred care. Person-centred care can be applied to any care situation, and four principles are associated with it; see Figure 43.1. For care to be enabling, there has to be a partnership between healthcare professionals and patients; they should work together, understanding what is important to the person, make decisions about their care and treatment, and identify and achieve their goals

Monitoring effectiveness

The Nursing Associate has a role to play in monitoring and measuring the effectiveness of care in partnership with people, their families and carers. There are a number of ways organisations (including regulators) can do this formally and informally, with questions such as is the patient's experience better, was the care better? and by seeking insight into what worked well with working in partnership and what worked less well and in what circumstances.

Observing at team meetings, undertaking in-depth interviews with participants and stakeholders, implementing an online survey of clinical teams and interviewing patient representatives can provide rich insight into efficacy. Monitoring draws on evidence from people using services and their families and advocates, staff as well as patient records (care plans).

The Nursing Associate is required to critically evaluate feedback from people, those they work with and relevant others to monitor and review the effectiveness of their practice.

Co-morbidities and holistic care provision

At the point of registration, the Nursing Associate will be able to: demonstrate an understanding of co-morbidities and the demands of meeting people's holistic needs when prioritising care.

Figure 44.1 An example of coordinated care for the elderly and those with complex needs.

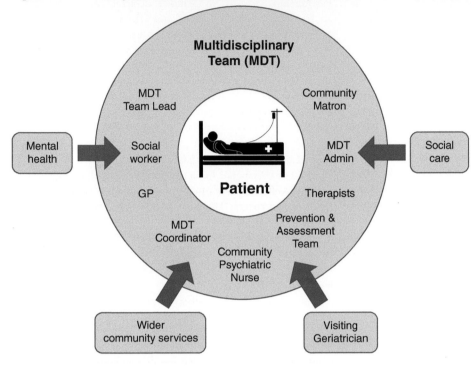

Top Tip

A holistic approach should be taken which recognises people's lived experience and the range of barriers they encounter, rather than using tick-box approaches to addressing barriers.

The Nursing Associate at a Glance, First Edition. Ian Peate.

As a Nursing Associate, you have to be able to understand co-morbidities and the demands of meeting people's holistic needs when planning and prioritising care. This requires a coordination of processes that will involve the planning and managing of safe discharge or transfer of patients between health and social care settings.

Addressing co-morbidities and the demands of meeting people's holistic needs when prioritising care means you will need to understand patient and public involvement and consistently demonstrate the principle of 'nothing about us without us' in all interactions with patients and carers. You will acknowledge the importance of making decisions with patients based on their wishes, as opposed to your or the organisation's wishes (see Chapter 43).

Co-morbidities

There is no agreement on the meaning of the term co-morbidity. Co-morbidity is associated with worse health outcomes, more complex clinical management and an increase in healthcare costs. There are some people who have a range of diagnoses and as such can have multiple and complex needs. A greater proportion of older people (compared to younger people) may require an interdisciplinary approach to their care so as to manage complex co-morbidities, social and psychological issues. The Nursing Associate needs to ensure that they have specific knowledge about care requirements and the right tools and skills to appropriately manage care. Those with complex care needs and co-morbidities will require a holistic, problem-solving approach to their care.

In general, co-morbidity refers to the presence of more than one disorder in the same person. For example, if a person is diagnosed with both general anxiety disorder and a major depressive disorder, that person could be said to have a co-morbid (coexisting) disorder. There are other conditions that are seen to overlap, and these can include physical disorders such as diabetes mellitus, cardiovascular disease, cancer, infectious diseases and dementia. Some mental health disorders that exhibit co-morbidity include eating disorders, anxiety disorders and substance use. Co-morbidity is associated with the presence of multiple mental or physical illnesses in the same person.

Holistic assessment

The team (hospital or primary care), in partnership with the patient, should be responsible for undertaking a holistic assessment of the patient, taking into consideration factors such as social support and if applicable employment as well as medical risks and needs. The assessment should be multidisciplinary so that professionals and patients are aware of any co-morbidities and can make referrals for further investigation and treatment if needed.

Co-morbidities are also common between physical long-term conditions. For example, people with arthritis are twice as likely to suffer from obesity or heart disease as people in the general population, and people with diabetes are at increased risk of stroke.

The impact of multi-morbidity is profound and multi-faceted. Those with several long-term conditions have poorer quality of life, poorer clinical outcomes, longer hospital stays and more post-operative complications. People with diabetes and co-morbidities show poorer adherence to treatment, experience more complications and use more medical care relative to those with diabetes alone.

Holistic care

When delivering holistic care and prioritising care for those with co-morbidities, assessments should be carried out to identify problems arising from the presence of several chronic conditions that are occurring together. Comprehensive assessment must involve listening to the patients' story and ensuring that their own personal goals are incorporated alongside those that have been identified clinically. To reiterate, being person-centred is critical to looking after those with multiple chronic illnesses, with an emphasis on including all aspects of their health, from physical to emotional and social well-being, so as to address their complex needs. See Figure 44.1 for an example of coordinated care for the elderly and those with complex needs.

Concerted efforts must be made to enhance continuity between some health and care services. Sometimes clinical pathways are not always joined up and are not consistent when patients move from primary to secondary care and back. The role of the Nursing Associate is key here to ensure prioritising of needs and the coordination of care between multidisciplinary teams for people with co-morbidities.

45 Capacity: understanding information and making decisions

At the point of registration, the Nursing Associate will be able to: recognise how a person's capacity affects their ability to make decisions about their own care and to give or withhold consent.

Section 2 of the Mental Capacity Act 2005 notes that 'a person lacks capacity in relation to a matter if at the material time he is unable to make a decision for himself in relation to the matter because of an impairment of, or a disturbance in the functioning of, the mind or brain'.

Box 45.1 The Mental Capacity Act 2005.

Lacking capacity includes where the ability to make decisions is affected permanently or in the short term:

- Permanently: The ability to make decisions is always affected. This could be because the person, has a form of dementia, a learning disability or brain injury.
- Short term: The ability to make decisions changes from day to day. This could be because the person is confused as a result of their medication, due to some mental health conditions, or if they are unconscious.

Box 45.2 Examples of permanent and short-term lack of capacity.

1 Paula has dementia; this impacts her short-term memory. When Paula has been shopping (spending money), she often forgets what she has purchased, or even if she has been shopping and also how much she has spent. It is doubtful that Paula's condition will improve in the future.
   Paula's capacity to make these important financial decisions has, in this case, been permanently affected as a result of her mental health condition.
2 Ranjit was involved in a road traffic collision. Usually, he has the capacity to carry out the activities of living unaided. However, as result of the road traffic collision, Ranjit is semi-conscious and in the short term he cannot attend to his activities of living unaided. His condition is likely to change from day to day.

Box 45.3 Assessing capacity.

- Before treatment, the Mental Capacity Act requires an assessment of a patient's capacity.
- Capacity is time and decision specific; therefore, assess a patient's ability to make a specific decision at the time the decision needs to be made.
- Never decide that someone lacks capacity based solely on age, appearance, condition or behaviour.
- A person's inability to make a major or complex decision does not mean that the person cannot make a smaller or simpler decision.

Box 45.4 The five key principles embodied in the Mental Capacity Act.

Principle 1: The presumption of capacity
Principle 2: Support the individual
Principle 3: Unwise decision
Principle 4: Best interests
Principle 5: Least restrictive option

Top Tip
A person's capacity to consent can change; they may have the capacity to make some decisions but not others, or their capacity may come and go.

The Nursing Associate at a Glance, First Edition. Ian Peate.
© 2021 John Wiley & Sons Ltd. Published 2021 by John Wiley & Sons Ltd.

When a person cannot make decisions for themselves because they do not have the mental capacity to make them, the Mental Capacity Act 2005 informs what can be done to plan ahead, how someone else can make decisions for the person and who can make decisions for the person if they have not planned ahead. See Box 45.1. The principles are outlined in this chapter

Capacity

Capacity refers to the ability of a person to understand information and make decisions. It can also sometimes mean the ability to communicate decisions about a person's life. If a person does not understand the information and is unable to make a decision about their treatment, they are said to lack capacity to make decisions about treatment. Lacking capacity can be short term and permanent; see Box 45.2.

There are different types of decisions to be made that will require different types of capacity. It would be expected that a lower level of mental capacity would be required to make decisions about everyday matters, for example, what kind of clothes to wear, what to eat.

A higher level of mental capacity would be needed if the person was making higher-level decisions, such as deciding on making a financial investment or giving consent for surgery.

Assessing capacity

The assessment of capacity is set out in the Mental Capacity Act 2005 and its Code of Practice (see Box 45.3). In order to determine or to assess a person's ability to make a decision, these questions should be asked, can the person:

- Understand the information related to the decision?
- Remember the information for long enough to make a decision?
- Weigh up or use the information to reach a decision?
- Communicate the decision in any way at all, for example, by talking, using sign language or hand signals, or squeezing a hand?

There are five key principles embodied in the Mental Capacity Act (see Box 45.4). The first of the three principles can help to help determine if a patient lacks capacity. If this is the case, then the remaining two principles are used to support the decision-making process.

Principles

Principle 1: The presumption of capacity

- Capacity should be assumed unless proved otherwise.
- Never assume someone is unable to make a decision based on medical condition or disability.

Principle 2: Support the individual

- Patients should be given all practicable help before they are deemed unable to make their own decisions.
- Make every effort to support a patient in making a specific decision for themselves if possible (they may need an advocate or a translator).
- Even if it has been established that the patient lacks capacity, always involve them as far as possible in making their decision.

Principle 3: Unwise decision

- Patients have the right to make decisions that you might disagree with or consider irrational or unwise.
- This does not imply a lack of capacity; it may reflect individual preferences or values.
- The ability to make the decision is central; not the decision itself.

Principle 4: Best interests

- Decisions made or action taken for or on behalf of a person who lacks mental capacity must be done in their best interests.
- 'Best interests' depends on individual circumstances, including the person's welfare, social, emotional and psychological interests and also their medical interests.
- Give consideration to the patient's current or previous wishes and their beliefs and values.

Principle 5: Least restrictive option

- If making a decision on behalf of a person lacking capacity, consider whether it is possible to delay the decision until the person regains capacity.
- If a decision is needed, consider if this can be done while interfering with the person's rights or freedoms as little as possible.
- If a person is temporarily incapacitated and the decision can be deferred until they regain capacity, do so.
- If this is not possible, make the decision in the person's best interests. The least restrictive option has to be considered wherever possible.

46 Self-harm and suicide

At the point of registration, the Nursing Associate will be able to: recognise people at risk of abuse, self-harm and/or suicidal ideation and the situations that may put them and others at risk.

Table 46.1 Risk factors (Source: WHO, 2014).

Societal	• Difficulties accessing or receiving care • Access to means of suicide • Inappropriate media reporting • Stigma associated with mental health, substance abuse or suicidal behaviour preventing people from seeking help
Community	• Poverty • Experiences of trauma or abuse • Experiences of disaster, war, or conflict • Experiences of discrimination
Relationships	• Isolation and lack of social support • Relationship breakdown • Loss or conflict
Individual	• Previous suicide attempts • Self-harm behaviours • Mental ill-health • Drug and alcohol misuse

Table 46.2 Protective factors.

Societal	• Easily accessible effective mental health support and treatment when needed
Community	• Being in full-time employment • Having supportive school environments for children and young people
Relationships	• Having strong and supportive social connections (for example, positive relationships with family, friends, partners)
Individual	• Problem-solving skills and coping skills that help people to manage in difficult circumstances • Feeling hopeful or optimistic toward the future even during times of stress

Top Tip

When working together, local organisations can combine expertise and resources to implement a number of interventions to prevent suicide including addressing risk factors such as self-harm.

The Nursing Associate at a Glance, First Edition. Ian Peate.
© 2021 John Wiley & Sons Ltd. Published 2021 by John Wiley & Sons Ltd.

Suicide and self-harm are global public health issues that have devastating effects on families, friends and communities. They are a priority for anyone working in health and social care and can take place anywhere, anytime. It could be a student in a school, a detainee in a prison or a colleague or family member.

Definitions

Self-harm is a broad term used to describe the various things that people do to hurt themselves physically. It includes cutting or scratching the skin, burning/branding with cigarettes/lighters, scalding, overdose of tablets or other toxins, tying ligatures around the neck, punching oneself or other surfaces, banging limbs/head and hair pulling. Sometimes the term self-harm is used to describe behaviours that may be culturally acceptable but, lead to self-inflicted physical or psychological damage, for example, smoking, recreational drug use, excessive alcohol or body enhancement. Self-harm is understood as physical injury inflicted as a means of managing an extreme emotional state – it can be life-saving or self-destructive. Suicide and suicidal behaviour are terms that refer to a deliberate act that is intended to end one's life.

Suicidal ideation

Suicidal ideation means wanting to take your own life or thinking about suicide. Passive suicidal ideation occurs a person wishes they were dead or that they could die, but they do not actually have any plans to commit suicide. Active suicidal ideation is not only thinking about it, but having the intent to commit suicide, including planning how to do it

Suicide

Each year in the UK thousands of people end their lives by suicide.

Suicide and suicide attempts may have lasting effects on individuals, their social networks and communities. The causes of suicide are varied, and the Nursing Associate has to understand the psychological processes that can result in suicidal thoughts and the factors that can lead to feelings of hopelessness or despair.

It must be acknowledged that suicide behaviours are complex, with no one single explanation of why people die by suicide. Social, psychological and cultural factors may all interact to lead a person to have suicidal thoughts or behaviour. A number of risk factors commonly come together to increase vulnerability to suicidal behaviour (see Table 46.1).

As well as risk factors, protective factors have also been identified. Protective factors are factors that could help to reduce vulnerability to suicidal behaviour. Considering how best to support and enhance people's access to protective factors is a key aspect of preventing suicide (see Table 46.2). ·

Self-harm

People may worry about the reaction of the Nursing Associate and the effect that it could have on relationships with family and friends. This can prevent them from seeking help. There may be a fear of being labelled an 'attention seeker' or bothering others around them. They may feel their concerns could be dismissed.

Some people who self-harm do so in a controlled way; for example, they do not cut deeply or harm themselves in a way that requires medical assistance. It is important to appreciate that as with all maladaptive coping strategies, self-harm may develop into a usual response to daily stresses and may escalate in severity.

It is essential to consider risk, as there are situations or factors that increase the level of potential risk to a person's safety. It is important to develop an understanding of the level of risk and appreciate that it can change over time, as the meaning or intent may change depending on the person's mood or circumstances.

Factors that may increase risk related to self-harm include:

- The use of alcohol or drugs when self-harming can make a person more reckless and impulsive.
- Feelings of hopelessness about life. This may lead to the person not caring whether they harm themselves, or they may actively want to die.
- Means of self-harm, where there is a higher risk of accidental or unanticipated severe harm. For example, frequent small overdoses can cause long-term harm.
- An increase in frequency of self-harm or a feeling that the person has to do more harm to feel the benefits.

Nursing Associates working in various settings, including the emergency department, schools, primary care, children's and young people's wards and acute medical wards, need to be alert to signs of self-harm.

47 Sharing information

At the point of registration, the Nursing Associate will be able to: take personal responsibility to ensure that relevant information is shared according to local policy and appropriate immediate action is taken to provide adequate safeguarding and that concerns are escalated.

Figure 47.1 When and how to share information (Source: HM Government 2018).

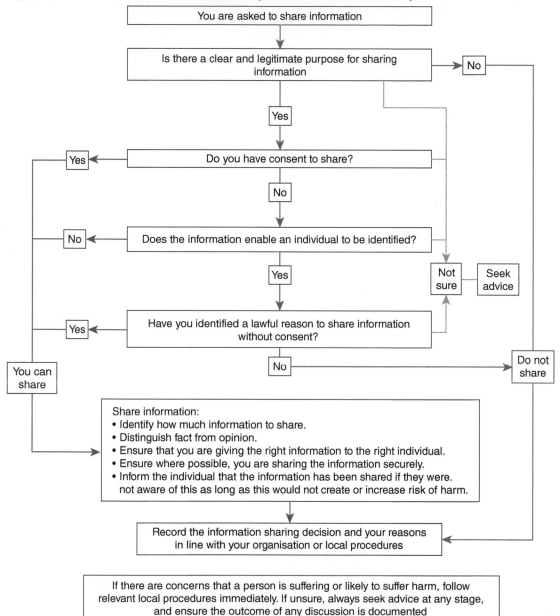

Top Tip

Information sharing is essential for effective safeguarding and promoting the welfare of people. Nursing Associates must have due regard to the relevant data protection principles that permit them to share personal information.

General Data Protection Regulation, Data Protection Act 208 and Human Rights Act

The General Data Protection Regulation (GDPR) apply to the health and care sectors across the UK. Under these regulations, patients have more control over their personal data, and organisations that use personal data are accountable for its lawful use and protection. The aim of the GDPR is to protect citizens from data breaches and protect privacy in a data-driven world. It applies to all companies that process personal data, particularly around access to it and control over how information is used.

The Data Protection Act 2018 balances the rights of the individual whom the information is about and the possible need to share information about them. Do not assume that sharing is prohibited; it is important to consider this balance in every case. Always keep a record of what has been shared.

As well as the GDPR and Data Protection Act 2018, Nursing Associates need also to balance the common law duty of confidence and the rights enshrined within the Human Rights Act 1998 against the effect on patients or individuals at risk if they do not share the information.

Sharing information

Nursing Associates and other health and social care professionals often have to make case-by-case decisions on the personal patient information they should give to other practitioners so as to ensure that the patient receives the right care and support, at the right time. The overall aim of information sharing is to improve outcomes for all. Information sharing and collaborative working can help to provide a more complete picture of an individual's needs, allowing for earlier and more effective intervention. This can then lead to faster and more coordinated delivery of services, which improves the patient experience. There are seven golden rules associated with sharing of information, and the Nursing Associate must take personal responsibility, ensuring that all relevant information is shared according to local policy and immediate appropriate action is taken to provide adequate safeguards and that concerns are escalated:

1 GDPR, Data Protection Act 2018 and human rights law are not barriers to justified information sharing; they provide a framework to ensure that personal information about living individuals is shared appropriately.

2 Be open and honest with the individual (and where appropriate, their family) from the outset regarding why, what, how and with whom information will, or might be shared. Seek their agreement, unless it is unsafe or inappropriate to do so.

3 Ask for advice from other practitioners, or the information governance lead, if in any doubt about sharing the information concerned and where possible without disclosing the identity of the individual.

4 Where possible, share information with consent, and respect the wishes of those who do not consent. GDPR and Data Protection Act 2018 notes that information may be shared without consent if, in your judgement, there is a lawful basis to do so, where safety may be at risk. Judgement must be based on the facts of the case.

5 Consider safety and well-being: Base information-sharing decisions on considerations of the safety and well-being of the individual and others who may be affected by their actions.

6 Ensure that the information shared is necessary, proportionate, relevant, adequate, accurate, timely and secure

7 Keep a record of decisions made and the reasons for it – whether it is to share information or not. Record what has been shared, with whom and for what purpose.

See Figure 47.1 for a flowchart that describes when and how to share information. Escalating concerns has been discussed in Chapter 31.

Consent

When consent is being gained in order to share information, this must always be unambiguous and freely given (without coercion). Also, consent may be withdrawn at any point. Wherever possible, seek consent and be open and honest with the individual from the outset. Always seek consent where an individual may not expect information to be passed on. There may, however, be some situations where it is not appropriate to seek consent. This may be because the individual cannot give consent, it is not reasonable to obtain consent, or because gaining consent would put a person's safety or well-being at risk. Where a decision has been made to share information without consent, a record of what has been shared should be kept, and local policy and procedure must be adhered to.

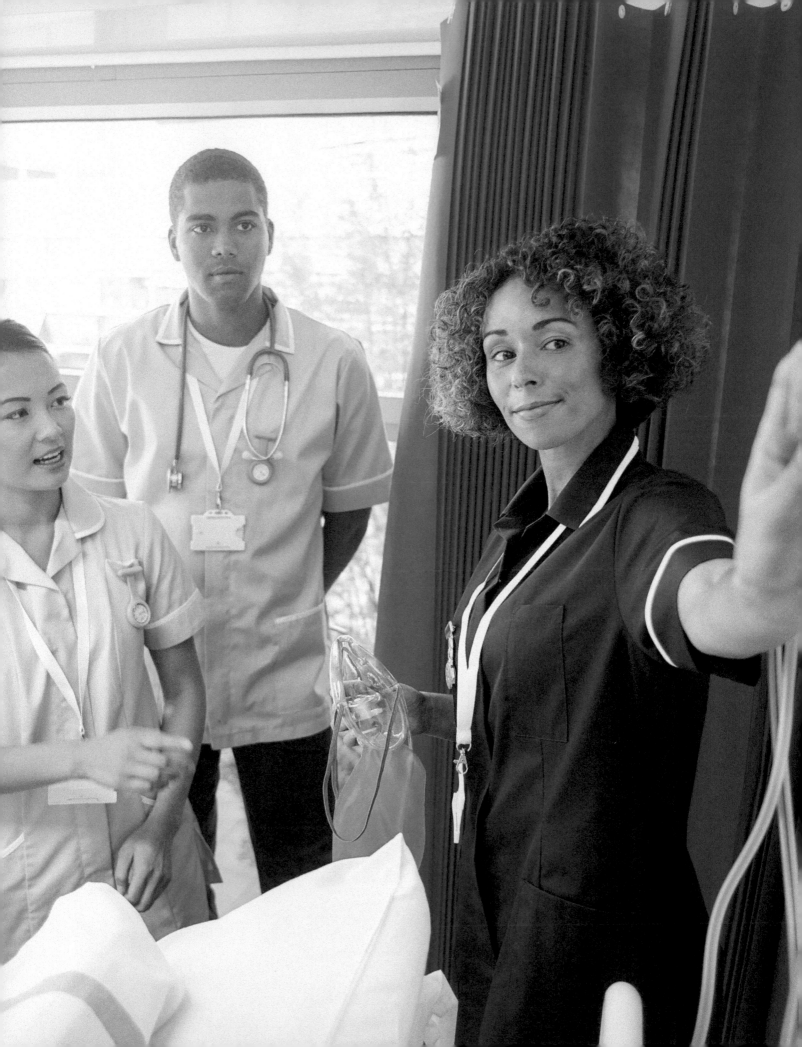

Working in teams

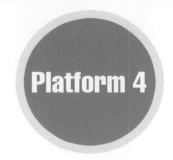

Platform 4

Chapters

48 Roles and responsibilities

At the point of registration, the Nursing Associate will be able to: demonstrate an awareness of the roles, responsibilities and scope of practice of different members of the nursing and interdisciplinary team, and their own role within it.

Table 48.1 Key differences between the roles of Nursing Associate and Registered Nurse (Source: NMC, 2019a).

Nursing Associate	Registered Nurse
Be an accountable professional	Be an accountable professional
Promoting health and preventing ill health	Promoting health and preventing ill health
Provide and monitor care	Provide and evaluate care
Working in teams	Leading and managing nursing care and working in teams
Improving safety and quality of care	Improving safety and quality of care
Contributing to integrated care	Coordinating care
	Assessing needs and planning care

Figure 48.1 Components of revalidation (Source: NMC, 2019b).

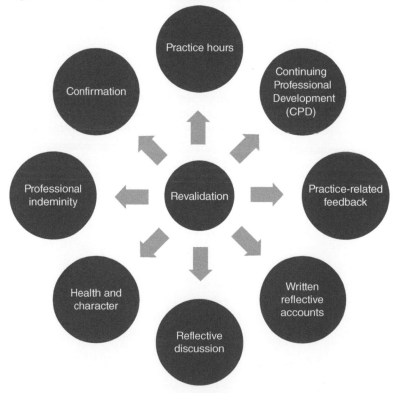

Top Tip

As is the case with nurses and other health professionals, Nursing Associates can expand their knowledge and skills with the right education and clinical governance

The Nursing Associate at a Glance, First Edition. Ian Peate.
© 2021 John Wiley & Sons Ltd. Published 2021 by John Wiley & Sons Ltd.

Nursing Associates have an active role to play as members of interdisciplinary teams. They are required to collaborate and communicate effectively with nurses, a variety of other health and care professionals, and a range of non-statutory carers. See also Chapter 63.

Nursing Associates

In England, Nursing Associates are a part of the nursing team, and the role was designed to help bridge the gap between health and care assistants and Registered Nurses. Nursing Associate, a protected title in law, is a stand-alone role that also provides a progression route into graduate-level nursing. Nursing Associates work with people of all ages and in a range of settings in health and social care.

The Nursing and Midwifery Council (NMC) have produced standards for the Nursing Associate and programmes they undertake, enabling them to join the professional register. Upon registration, the Nursing Associate must demonstrate that they have the skills required to care for people safely, with integrity, expertise, respect and compassion.

Nursing Associates play a part in most aspects of care, including delivery and monitoring. Registered Nurses take the lead on assessment, planning and evaluation. They lead on managing and coordinating care with full input from the Nursing Associate as a member of the integrated care team. Key differences between the roles of Nursing Associate and Registered Nurse are identified in Table 48.1.

Scope of practice

This can be defined as the range of roles, functions, responsibilities and activities which the Nursing Associate is educated, deemed proficient and authorised to perform. The Nursing Associate may expand their scope of practice, within the regulatory framework, through further education and experience after joining the professional register.

How the Nursing Associate performs their range of roles is influenced by the guiding values and principles regarding how nursing practice is provided, for example, the Code of Professional Conduct. The scope of practice is dynamic, and changes as the Nursing Associate progresses in their career. It must also respond to the ever-changing needs of the population and the health service.

Scope of practice lays out the procedures, actions and processes that the Nursing Associate performs. The individual practitioner's scope is determined by a range of factors that gives them the authority to perform a particular role or task. Decisions that are made about a Nursing Associate's scope of practice are complex, with a number of important determining factors that need to be considered including the values that underpin practice, levels of proficiency, an understanding of responsibility and accountability and the support and resources available. With each Nursing Associate being responsible and accountable for their own scope of practice, responsibility and accountability are the cornerstone of contemporary practice.

Collaborative practice

Collaboration with the interdisciplinary team – coming together to deliver the highest quality of care – will also impact the scope of practice. Interdisciplinary working demonstrates a professional attitude and acceptance of responsibility for the individual's practice (see also Chapter 49).

An essential component of collaborative practice is the professional relationship between the Nursing Associate and other healthcare professionals. Collaborative practice entails respectful, effective communication and appropriate documentation. An understanding of the scope of practice underpins collaborative practice relationships. It is the responsibility of the Nursing Associate to inform other healthcare professionals about their own individual scope of practice.

Continuing professional development

Continuing professional development (CPD) contributes towards the development of all registrants. It is, therefore, a lifelong process made up of structured and informal learning taking place after the completion of initial registration. CPD is a legal requirement involving planned learning experiences designed to enhance knowledge, skills and attitudes.

The acquisition of new knowledge is essential if the Nursing Associate is to practise competently, confidently and effectively in constantly changing health and social care environments.

Nursing Associates are required to renew their registration every three years through the same revalidation process that applies to other registrants; see Figure 48.1 (see also Chapter 61).

49 Interacting with members of the care team

At the point of registration, the Nursing Associate will be able to: demonstrate an ability to support and motivate other members of the care team and interact confidently with them.

Figure 49.1   Some symptoms of emotional exhaustion.

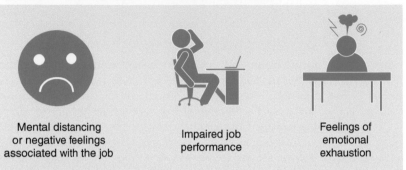

Mental distancing or negative feelings associated with the job

Impaired job performance

Feelings of emotional exhaustion

Top Tip

Motivated people have a positive outlook. They are excited about what they are doing. Also, they know that they are investing their time in something that is meaningful. Motivated people enjoy their work and perform well.

The Nursing Associate at a Glance, First Edition. Ian Peate.
© 2021 John Wiley & Sons Ltd. Published 2021 by John Wiley & Sons Ltd.

The Code of Professional Conduct

The importance of effective teamwork and interacting with members of the care team is highlighted in the Nursing and Midwifery Council's (NMC's) Professional Code. The Code makes it clear that the Nursing Associate must work in a cooperative manner. In order to accomplish this:

- Respect the skills, expertise and contributions of your colleagues, referring matters to them when appropriate.
- Maintain effective communication with colleagues.
- Keep colleagues informed when you are sharing the care of individuals with other health and care professionals and staff.
- Work with colleagues to evaluate the quality of your work and that of the team.
- Work with colleagues to ensure the safety of those receiving care.
- Share information to identify and reduce risk.
- Be supportive of colleagues who are encountering health or performance problems. However, this support must never compromise, or be at the expense of, patient or public safety.

Effective clinical practice focuses not only on the various technological systems, but also on human factors, which include professional communication and team collaboration. Human factors are as important as technology and help to prevent errors, promote patent safety and enhance care outcomes. See also Chapter 50.

We interact with many other people as we go about our work. The quality of these various interactions can have a significant effect on the health and well-being of the people we offer care and support to, and also on our own health and well-being and our enjoyment of work. The patient experience is often better when staff feel they have a good working environment; co-worker support; supervisor support as well as job satisfaction; a positive organisational culture; organisational support along with low emotional exhaustion.

Emotional exhaustion

Emotional exhaustion (sometimes referred to as burnout) results in a total system breakdown, after protracted, unmanageable stress and emotional fatigue. This can result in emotional, cognitive and physical exhaustion and may have serious physical- and mental-health-related consequences. It can take a long time and much treatment to recover from emotional exhaustion; see Figure 49.1.

It is in everyone's best interests to support and motivate other members of the care team and to interact in a confident manner with them.

Delegation

Delegation can be defined as directing another to carry out work or perform a duty. It is concerned with allowing a person to act on behalf of another. The duties of delegation can be seen as the process by which the delegator decides to allocate clinical or non-clinical treatment or care to a competent person. The person delegating will always remain responsible for the overall management of the patient and remains accountable for the original decision to delegate. It is important to note is that the delegator will not be accountable for the decisions and actions of the competent person (the delegatee).

The Nursing Associate must be accountable for their decisions to delegate tasks and duties to other people, and they must only delegate those tasks and duties that are within the other person's competence, ensure that those they delegate tasks to are effectively supervised and supported, and to confirm that the outcome of any task delegated to someone else has met the required standard.

The principles of delegation include:

- Delegation has to be, at all times, in the best interest of the patient.
- The person being delegated to must have been suitably trained to undertake the intervention.
- Full records of training given should be kept.
- Evidence that the support worker's competence has been assessed should be recorded.
- There should be clear guidelines and protocols in place.
- The role should be within the worker's job description.
- The team and any support staff need to be informed that the activity has been delegated.
- The person delegating the activity must ensure that an appropriate level of supervision and mentorship is available.
- The delegatee must undergo ongoing training to ensure that their competence is maintained.
- The whole process must be assessed to identify any risks.

50 Human factors and team working

At the point of registration, the Nursing Associate will be able to: understand and apply the principles of human factors and environmental factors when working in teams.

Table 50.1 Human and ergonomic factors (Source: https://www. pngfuel.com/free-png/dieha).

Human	We all have limitations (physical and mental).
Workplace	People are subjected to a high cognitive workload.
Environment	Relevant information is adopted in systems and work environment design.
Technologies	Technologies/systems that people are using have become complex.

Box 50.1 Some examples of never events (Source: Adapted NHS Improvement, 2018).

- Wrong site surgery
- Wrong implant/prosthesis
- Retained foreign object post-procedure
- Mis-selection of a strong potassium containing solution (medication)
- Wrong route of medication
- Overdose of insulin due to abbreviations or incorrect device
- Overdose of methotrexate for non-cancer treatment
- Failure to install functional collapsible shower or curtain rails (suicide risk)
- Falls from poorly restricted windows
- Chest or neck entrapment in bedrails
- Incompatible transfusion or transplantation
- Misplaced naso- or oro-gastric tubes
- Scalding of patients

Top Tip

Learning from what goes wrong in healthcare is key to avoiding future harm. This requires a culture of openness and honesty so that staff, patients, families and carers feel supported to speak up in a constructive way.

The Nursing Associate at a Glance, First Edition. Ian Peate.
© 2021 John Wiley & Sons Ltd. Published 2021 by John Wiley & Sons Ltd.

Chapter 49 of this text discusses the importance of effective interaction within teams and the importance of supporting and motivating other members of the care team and demonstrating the ability to engage confidently with them. This chapter will focus on human and environmental factors when working in teams.

The key purpose of any health and social care system is to deliver high-quality care to all. High-quality care means care that is safe, clinically effective and results in as positive an experience for patients as possible.

Human factors

Human factors (often referred to as ergonomics) include environmental/workplace, organisational and job factors and human and individual characteristics that have the potential to influence behaviour at work in a way that may affect health and safety (see Table 50.1). Clinical human factors/ergonomics is defined as enhancing clinical performance through an understanding of the effects of teamwork, tasks, equipment, workspace, culture and organisation on human behaviour and abilities and application of that knowledge in clinical settings.

Ergonomics is the study of the interaction between humans and manmade objects. It relates the person to the work that they do so that their performance can be improved.

Never events

Never events are wholly preventable events, where guidance or safety recommendations that provide strong systemic protective barriers are available at the national level and should have been implemented by all healthcare providers. Every never event type can cause serious patient harm or death. However, serious harm or death is not required to have occurred as a result of a specific incident occurrence for that incident to be categorised as a never event.

Learning from never events

When things go wrong in care, it is vital that they are recorded so as to ensure that learning can take place. Working out what has gone wrong and why it has gone wrong is necessary in order to put in place effective and sustainable actions that have to be taken to reduce the risk of similar incidents occurring again.

Incidents have to be reported in accordance with local policy and procedure, which is often the organisation's risk management system, where staff are encouraged to record details of incidents so that learning and service improvement may occur. Learning lessons from incidents requires timely incident reporting, which in turn requires a fair, open and just culture that rejects blame as a tool.

Health and care staff and the general public are encouraged to report patient safety incidents, whether they result in harm or not. Learning from what goes wrong in healthcare is crucial to preventing future harm, but it requires a culture of openness and honesty to ensure that staff, patients, families and carers feel supported to speak up in a constructive way. It is unacceptable for the Nursing Associate or any other member of staff to fail to report a never event. Some examples of never events can be found in Box 50.1.

The Nursing Associate's input

Human factors is a discipline that promotes user-centred design and a systems approach to safety. There are some human factors techniques and approaches that may require specialist input. However, the basic principles are often common sense and can be used to help improve safety. Patient safety is an integral aspect of nursing practice. It is part of everyday clinical practice. An understanding of clinical human factors will help the Nursing Associate appreciate how the design of the systems, processes, equipment and environment where they work enhances their ability and the ability of others to deliver safe patient care. This understanding or appreciation of human factors is essential if Nursing Associates are to make significant improvements in enhancing patient safety in clinical practice.

Nursing Associates and others who work closely with patients and carers will often have a unique view of what can and does go wrong; as such, this invaluable insight can be used to help find solutions.

51 Data management

At the point of registration, the Nursing Associate will be able to: demonstrate the ability to effectively and responsibly access, input, and apply information and data using a range of methods including digital technologies and share appropriately within interdisciplinary teams.

Figure 51.1 Potential benefits of sharing data.

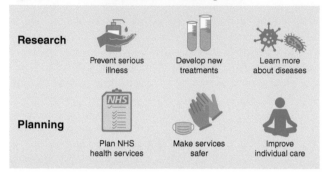

Research
- Prevent serious illness
- Develop new treatments
- Learn more about diseases

Planning
- Plan NHS health services
- Make services safer
- Improve individual care

Box 51.1 Some examples of functional areas as well as the format of the records.

Function:
- Patient health records (electronic or paper based, including those concerning all specialties and GP records)
- Records of private patients seen on NHS premises
- Emergency Department, birth, and all other registers
- Theatre registers and minor operations (and other related) registers
- Administrative records (including, for example, personnel, estates, financial and accounting records, notes associated with complaint-handling)
- X-ray and imaging reports, output and images
- Integrated health and social care records
- Data processed for secondary use purposes. Secondary use is any use of person level or aggregate level data that is not for direct care purposes. This can include data for service management, research or for supporting commissioning decisions.

Format:
- Photographs, slides, and other images
- Microform (i.e. microfiche/microfilm)
- Audio and video tapes, cassettes, CD-ROM, etc.
- E-mails
- Computerised records

Top Tip

Having access to the right information at the right time is key to supporting effective clinical decisions enabling the Nursing Associate to provide the right care for patients.

The Nursing Associate at a Glance, First Edition. Ian Peate.
© 2021 John Wiley & Sons Ltd. Published 2021 by John Wiley & Sons Ltd.

The constraints on and privileges associated with sharing of data have been discussed elsewhere in this text (for example, Chapter 47), where the principles of General Data Protection Regulation (GDPR) have been outlined. This chapter considers how the Nursing Associate (working with others) manages data using a range of technologies.

Data

What is data? We all use data every day both in our personal and professional lives. Tapping a card to pay for shopping, accessing the Internet to order a meal and scanning the QR code to read a menu are examples of how we use data in our personal lives.

Documentation is an essential part of the role of the Nursing Associate. It serves as a communication vehicle for the Nursing Associate and other healthcare providers to relate to the patient's [his]story. The information within the documentation can be highly complex. Data are at the heart of that documentation. Nursing Associates invest much time in compiling and adding to patient documentation depicting the patient care delivered. Summarising health and care data in a structured way is the cornerstone of accurate, reliable and clinically meaningful measurement in care settings. Data and quality of care go hand in hand. Using data consistently and reliably will also allow for information to be collected once and reused for multiple purposes, including outcomes measurement, practice-level improvements, surveillance, population health, research and decision support (see Figure 51.1).

Recording assessment data when using a computer keyboard represents just as much caring communication between the Nursing Associate and patients as writing it down on a form. The most important factor is not the mode of recording but the interpersonal skills and motivation of the Nursing Associate when gathering the assessment data.

The management of data and records (accessing and inputting data), regardless of data type, is subject to legal and local regulations. Box 51.1 gives examples of functional areas as well as the format of the records.

The Professional Record Standards Body (PRSB) and the electronic health record

The aim of the PRSB is to ensure that the structure and content of all electronic health records in health and social care adhere to widely agreed high-quality information standards so there is a single, comprehensive, useable electronic health record (EHR) regardless of care setting.

As health and social care providers make the change from paper-based systems to the EHR, many possibilities arise that enable organisations to collect important information. However, there is a need to protect the privacy and security of the data.

e-Health technologies

e-Health, according to the World Health Organization, is 'the cost-effective and secure use of information and communications technologies in support of health and health-related fields, including health care services, health surveillance, health literature, and health education, knowledge and research'.

Digital technologies are transforming the ways patients can be empowered to actively engage in their own care, with a greater focus on well-being, to prevent diseases such as cancer, diabetes, hypertension, to determine the most appropriate treatments and to customise the management of long-term conditions, such as schizophrenia, depression, diabetes and asthma.

More and more, medical data are being generated by patients that are then processed by computers. Using wearable wireless sensors, patients can use other devices (for example, the smartphone) to generate medical data, including measuring oxygen saturations and glucose levels, blood pressure and heart rhythm. There are also hi-tech medical imaging devices that are being developed to replace the stethoscope. The generation of patient data will continue so that it can be integrated and analysed, empowering individuals and populations. Technology can assist in extracting meaningful information, and when the data are tracked and analysed, trends can be identified.

52 Prioritising care and co-morbidities

At the point of registration, the Nursing Associate will be able to: demonstrate an understanding of co-morbidities and the demands of meeting people's holistic needs when prioritising care.

Figure 52.1 Two populations at risk of comorbidities across the life span (Source: Department of Health, ND).

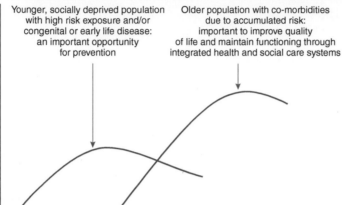

Risk of co-morbidity

Younger, socially deprived population with high risk exposure and/or congenital or early life disease: an important opportunity for prevention

Older population with co-morbidities due to accumulated risk: important to improve quality of life and maintain functioning through integrated health and social care systems

Age

Table 52.1 Six practical approaches to help develop care provision (Source: Adopted Bramley and Moody, 2016).

Think 'who could benefit'	Some people with multimorbidity may not need a tailored approach. Conversely, some people with a single but very complex LTC may benefit from it.
Think 'person-centred'	Begin by asking *'what matters to you?'* as opposed to *'what's the matter?'* This encourages a focus on person-centred care
Think 'planning'	A well-thought-out collaborative planning process is essential for people with multimorbidity, identifying what is most important to people.
Think 'mental and physical health'	Mental health and cognitive problems can be barriers to self-care and management of both physical and mental health conditions. These are important factors to consider when discussing care with the patient (and their carer).
Think 'Younger People too'	Although more common in older people, multimorbidity can also occur in younger people.
Think 'carer'	Informal carers, friends and family, will often provide considerable support to people with multimorbidity. Adopt an integrated approach to identifying and assessing carer health and well-being.

Top Tip

Caring for people with multimorbidity can be complicated as different conditions and their treatments often interact in complex ways.

Co-morbidities

Co-morbidities (also referred to multimorbidities, or multiple co-morbidities or multiple chronic conditions, multiple long-term conditions (LTCs)) are common and greatly increase the complexity of caring for people. They can be defined as the co-occurrence of two or more LTCs in a person. In addition, co-morbidities can be further defined as those that are clinically dominant, for example, where one illness outdoes another, where an index condition such as dementia overshadows the diagnosis or the treatment of another, for example, heart disease (known as diagnostic overshadowing); synergistic, related to the way in which they arise and are treated, such as chronic obstructive pulmonary disease and heart disease; and coincidental, where there are no obvious relationships, and the disease management is separate.

Targeted interventions

People with multiple LTCs are becoming the norm as opposed to the exception, and the number of people with co-morbidities is set to increase (see also Chapter 63 of this text).

It is important to identify specific populations that will require specific targeted interventions. There are at least two key populations with co-morbidities who will require a different emphasis of action: (1) those who have co-morbidities predominantly due to an increased life expectancy and as such a longer exposure to risk factors over time and (2) those who have co-morbidities primarily from more intense exposure to risk factors, particularly smoking, obesity, alcohol and physical inactivity as a result of challenging personal, occupational and societal factors throughout the person's life including persistent and widening inequalities (see Figure 52.1). Often these patients face complex physical, social and emotional problems and are more likely to have mental health difficulties. Prevention and action on the wider determinants is essential to improving life expectancy and well-being of this latter, younger group. However, strategies to maintain everyday functioning and quality of life through coordinated services are particularly important for the first group.

Shared decisions

Providing care for those with multimorbidity is complicated, because different conditions and their treatments very often interact in complex ways. The delivery of care for people with multiple LTCs should be built around individual conditions. The person should be seen both as a whole and as a part of any decision being made. When an individual-conditions approach is adopted care provision may be fragmented and may fail to take into account the combined impact of the conditions and their treatments on an individual's quality of life.

What is advocated is a bespoke approach so that people are put at the heart of decisions about their care. When this is in place, Nursing Associates and other health and social care professionals can offer their best advice and support. Skilled clinical judgement and effective communication are essential prerequisites when offering good care for people with multimorbidity.

Primary care

The UK has led modern primary care development, and many countries continue to look to the NHS as a model to emulate. However, primary and community care services now need to address increasing workloads, a population that is ageing and increasingly complex medical problems that are being diagnosed and managed in the community. General practice nurses are seeing patients with increasingly complex problems, some of whom are requiring longer face-to-face consultations.

The relationship between the public and health professionals is also changing, with an increased focus on providing people with information and ensuring that they are involved in decisions about their care. The Nursing Associate is key to addressing the challenge that those with multiple morbidities face as well as the challenges that services face.

Primary care is changing, with an increasing focus on the GP practice holding responsibility for the care of its registered patients. Many healthcare professionals will be required to develop new roles. More often, patients will be seen by new types of healthcare professionals, and there is a need for primary care practice to include a wider range of disciplines. The methods healthcare providers use to communicate with patients and with other health professionals will need to develop further, using a range of technologies including electronic messaging and videoconferencing.

53 Giving and receiving constructive feedback

At the point of registration, the Nursing Associate will be able to: demonstrate the ability to monitor and review the quality of care delivered, providing challenge and constructive feedback, when an aspect of care has been delegated to others.

Table 53.1 Some types of feedback.

Type	Discussion
Informal	Informal feedback is the most frequent form, provided on a day-to-day basis, given on any aspect of a Nursing Associate's professional performance and conduct. It can be given by any member of the multidisciplinary team. It can be seen as an opportunity to let someone know that you appreciate their efforts. For example, this could be at the end of a challenging shift on the ward or a chance meeting in a corridor. Often it is in verbal form.
Formal	This type of feedback comes as part of structured, planned assessment. Examples can include appraisals, discussions after a particular piece of work has been undertaken and feedback provided after an unsuccessful job interview. Any member of the multidisciplinary team can offer it. It is most often used by supervisors, peers or superiors. Often it is given in written format.
Formative	Formative feedback, 'for learning', is about a learner's progress at a particular time through a course or during the acquisition of a new skill. It provides opportunities to gain feedback, reflect and redirect effort (where appropriate) before completing a final assessment. It provides the opportunity of writing or performing a task without it having a direct impact on formal progress, and relies on continuous encouragement.
Summative	Summative feedback, 'of learning', measures performance, often against a standard, and comes with a mark/grade and feedback to explain the mark. It can be used to rank or judge an individual's performance.

Figure 53.1 Situation, behaviour, impact (Source: Mind Tools, 2017).

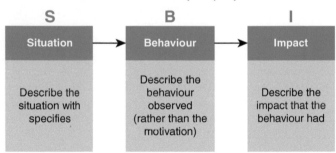

Situation-Behaviour-Impact (SBI) Model

Top Tip

Developing respectful and robust professional relationships are preconditions for giving/receiving constructive feedback acting as an influential motivator. All humans want to be validated and appreciated.

hapter 49 of this text considers the delegation of care to others. It should be reiterated here that if the Nursing Associate delegates care to another person (the delegatee) the Nursing Associate will always remain responsible for the overall management of the patient and will remain accountable for the original decision made to delegate.

Feedback

When we give feedback, we offer our opinions or evaluations of someone else's behaviour or performance. Giving and receiving feedback is not always an easy activity, and it can sometimes bring with it significant challenges for both the person giving and for the person receiving feedback. Giving and receiving effective feedback are skills that the Nursing Associate must develop and hone. They are key requirements in any contemporary healthcare settings. The process is inextricably linked to professional development and improved performance, both of which impact the quality of health and care services as well as patient satisfaction. Providing constructive feedback means focusing on behaviours that can be improved. Respectful and robust professional relationships are prerequisites for giving/receiving constructive feedback. Table 53.1 outlines some types of feedback

Being able to competently provide constructive feedback is an essential skill that the Nursing Associate needs. It is the basis of relationships, as well as being a part of the professional peer review process. When feedback is delivered well, the person receiving the feedback is motivated to improve their performance and to achieve desired outcomes.

Positive feedback can act as reinforcement, strengthening the likelihood of the desired behaviour continuing. It can guide and also suggest ways to improve performance.

The opposite can occur when feedback is delivered is a callous and harsh manner. The other person can then feel anger and resentment, all of which can impact care delivery and the person's self-esteem.

How to give feedback

Feedback should always be given in a timely manner, as soon after the event as possible. There are no right ways to give effective feedback. There are, however, a number of feedback models available that may help. The approach used will very much depend on the person receiving the feedback and also on the situation.

The Feedback Sandwich

The feedback sandwich aims to reduce any detrimental effect the negative feedback may have on the person; the aim is to encourage, not to discourage. This approach comprises three components:

1 Start off with positive feedback.
2 Introduce constructive or negative feedback.
3 Close with specific feedback that can build up trust and comfort.

Situation, behaviour, impact feedback tool

This tool offers the person the opportunity to reflect more on their actions whilst appreciating what you are commenting on and why, as well as what needs to change. The person gets the opportunity to reflect on the situation from another perspective as well as a chance to discuss strategies required for improvement with you (see Figure 53.1).

1 Begin by identifying the situation that the feedback is referring to.
2 Next define the specific behaviours you want to address.
3 Finally, end by describing how the person's behaviours impacted you or others.

Pendleton's Model of Feedback

Pendleton's model of feedback (Pendleton et al. 1984) helps make the experience being discussed constructive by:

1 Highlighting positive behaviours
2 Reinforcing these behaviours and including a discussion of the skills required to achieve them
3 Discussing what the person could have done differently.

Areas of improvement are first identified, and then they are followed up with a discussion about strategies that are required to improve performance.

Think about where to give feedback. Giving feedback loudly in a noisy corridor, or in the presence of others, is inappropriate. In this manner, the objectivity of the feedback will be lost, and the recipient may consider it as offensive. This may impact their professional relationship with peers and patients.

After delivering the feedback, remember to send a written summary of the session and to follow up on what has been discussed.

54 Role modelling

At the point of registration, the Nursing Associate will be able to: support, supervise and act as a role model to Nursing Associate students, healthcare support workers and those new to care roles, review the quality of the care they provide, promoting reflection and providing constructive feedback.

Box 54.1 The assessment process.

The assessment process usually involves the following stages:

- Prior to placement, the Trainee Nursing Associate makes contact with placement
- Induction (placement orientation)
- Initial meeting/interview (learning and development needs are identified)
- Formulation of learning contracts and action plans
- Midpoint meeting/interview (progress is discussed and other learning and development needs are identified)
- Feedback on professional values assessment
- Reflection on service user views
- Service users' contribution to assessment
- Formative assessment
- Final meeting/interview (progress and achievement explored) and summative assessment.

Figure 54.1 The practice assessment relationship.

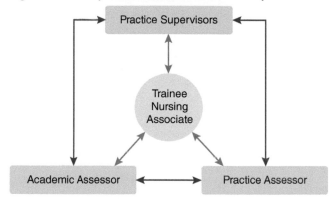

Top Tip
Role modelling is an import approach to transmitting positive values and attitudes.

Reflective practice has been discussed in Chapter 15 of this text, emphasising how important this activity is in enabling the Nursing Associate to make sense of events, situations and actions occurring in the workplace.

The Code requires the Nursing Associate to act as a role model of professional behaviour for students and newly qualified Nurses, Midwives and Nursing Associates to aspire to.

Role models

Role models can be described as those people with whom we identify, those who have certain qualities that we would like to have, are in positions we would like to reach or demonstrate behaviours and attitudes that others wish to copy.

Role models can inspire others and create a culture that supports and empowers staff to contribute to safe and effective person-centred care. The role model acts as a facilitator and manager of change. They influence others when needed. Role models enjoy nursing, are professionally competent and provide excellent patient care. They lead by example, interact with Trainee Nursing Associates, enjoy teaching and demonstrating clinical skills and have a caring attitude.

How a person will feel and how they fit into a new work environment can be influenced by how others behave. This can often be a stressful time for the new member of staff. How the Nursing Associate welcomes a new member of staff or Trainee Nursing Associate can have a powerful impact. Consider the qualities and behaviours you are exhibiting, and how these can impact others. Take time to reflect on those behaviours. How do you communicate with others? How cooperative are you? How do you demonstrate compassion, honesty and integrity? Are you striving for high standards and setting the benchmark for others to copy?

Supporting and supervising others

The Nursing and Midwifery Council (NMC) have published standards for supervision and assessment of students (this includes Trainee Nursing Associates). In these standards, they state that Nursing Associates may act as Practice Supervisors for Student Nurses so long as this is within the scope of their practice. They can also act as Practice Assessors for Trainee Nursing Associates.

Health Education England have produced a template in collaboration with stakeholders that is used by universities and placement providers detailing practice assessment requirements.

Supervising and assessing: Nursing Associates

Practice supervision enables students to learn and safely achieve proficiency and autonomy in their professional role. All NMC-registered Nurses, Midwives and Nursing Associates are able to supervise students, acting as role models for safe and effective practice.

Practice supervision

Practice supervision helps students to learn and safely achieve proficiency and autonomy in their professional role. Trainee Nursing Associates can be supervised by other registered health and social care professionals.

Practice assessment

Assessments and confirmation of proficiency rely on an understanding of student achievements in both theory and practice. Practice Assessors are required to make and record objective, evidence-based assessments that are grounded on conduct, proficiency and achievement, drawing on student records, direct observations, student self-reflection, as well as other resources. The nominated Practice Assessor works in partnership with a nominated Academic Assessor to evaluate and recommend the student for progression for each part of the programme. See Box 54.1.

As the NMC standards are implemented, the traditional model of mentorship changes. The role of mentors and sign-off mentors are to be replaced by Practice Supervisors, Practice Assessors and Academic Assessors. See Figure 54.1 for an example of how this relationship works.

The Trainee Nursing Associate is continually assessed based on the person's achievement of proficiency. Each Nursing Associate programme will have its own processes, and there are assessment criteria for each part of the programme indicating the expected levels of achievement. The proficiencies achieved within each part of the programme will also reflect expectations of personal and professional development.

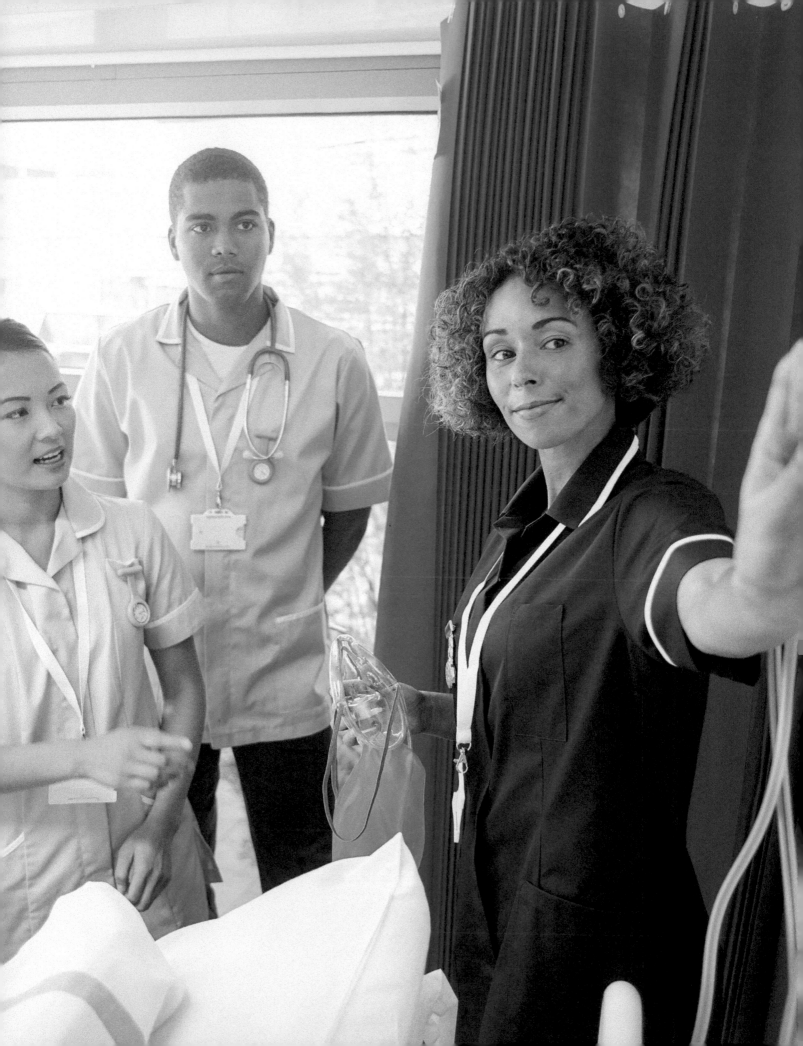

Improving safety and quality of care

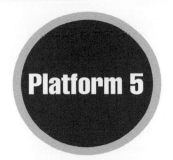

Platform 5

Chapters

55 Health and safety legislation

At the point of registration, the Nursing Associate will be able to: understand and apply the principles of health and safety legislation and regulations and maintain safe work and care environments.

Box 55.1 Legislation.

Health and Safety at Work etc. Act 1974
Management of Health and Safety at Work Regulations 1999
Workplace (Health, Safety and Welfare) Regulations 1992
The Health and Safety (Display Screen Equipment) Regulations 1992
The Manual Handling Operations Regulations 1992 amended 2002
The Regulatory Reform (Fire Safety) Order 2005
RIDDOR (Reporting of Injuries, Diseases and Dangerous
  Occurrences Regulations 1995)
The Personal Protective Equipment at Work Regulations 1992
COSHH (Control of Substances Hazardous to Health) 2002
The Provision and Use of Work Equipment Regulations 1998 (PUWER)
The Working Time Regulations 1998

Box 55.2 Risk assessment (see also Box 55.3).

- Walking round the environment identifying and taking notes of the hazards seen
- Determine who is most at risk from these hazards
- Evaluating the risks from the hazards, with decisions being made on whether existing safety policies and procedures are sufficient
- Identifying ways of removing the hazards
- Compiling a report on the findings

Table 55.1 Three steps to the identification of risk assessment.

Spot the hazard	Assess the risk	Make the changes
A hazard is anything that could hurt you or someone else	Work out how likely it is that the hazard will hurt someone and how badly they could be hurt	Eliminate, substitute, isolate, add safeguards, use safest procedure and use protective equipment

Box 55.3 The mnemonic RISKS.

- **R**egularly look for hazards
- **I**dentify those most at risk
- **S**ee whether current policies are protective enough
- **K**eep the area hazard-free
- **S**hare findings with your manager

Top Tip

The Health and Safety at Work etc Act 1974 and other regulations are legal requirements, they are not a matter of choice.

The Nursing Associate at a Glance, First Edition. Ian Peate.
© 2021 John Wiley & Sons Ltd. Published 2021 by John Wiley & Sons Ltd.

It is not possible for people to remain healthy if they are working or being cared for in environments that are unhealthy and unsafe. Looking after the workplace falls to all of us (employees and employers), promoting workplace health as we look after others, be these the patients we offer care to, people we visit in their homes and those colleagues we work with.

Healthy and safe workplaces, the right environments, are essential if patients are to make a recovery and become well. This is also important for healthcare workers to be able to perform their work activities safely and effectively.

The workplace can pose a number of dangers, and all employers have a responsibility to undertake risk assessments to identify the measures that need to be taken to protect staff and visitors from hazards. An assessment has to be undertaken and recorded where there are more than five people in the organisation.

Legislation

The key pieces of legislation that deal with a variety of aspects of health and safety are the Health and Safety at Work, etc. Act 1974 as well as the Management of Health and Safety at Work Regulations 1999. These two acts set the standards for all health and safety in the UK workplace. There are also secondary aspects of health and safety legislation that are more focussed, more specific and address a range of subjects, for example, manual handling, fire and display screen equipment. When all of these are brought together, they form the legal framework for health and safety in the workplace. See Box 55.1.

Risk assessment

In health and safety, a hazard is considered anything with the potential to cause harm. The hazard may not have harmed anyone yet; however, if it could cause harm, then it is a hazard.

There are three steps to the identification of risk assessment (see Table 55.1): spotting the hazard (hazard identification), assessing the risk (risk assessment) (Box 55.2) and making the changes (risk control).

A risk assessment highlights the risks and hazards in the workplace that could cause harm to patients, visitors and staff.

The law requires employers to conduct risk assessments of their workplaces. The employee also has responsibilities. They are required be vigilant and on the lookout for hazards, and to take action to resolve them when they are identified. The mnemonic RISKS (see Box 55.3) can help when undertaking a risk assessment.

Hazards

Spotting the hazard – The Nursing Associate must remain alert to anything that could be dangerous. If you see, hear or smell anything of concern, take note and report this. If this could be a hazard, then inform your manager, tell someone.

Assessing the risk – Determine how likely it is that a hazard will harm someone and how serious the harm might be. Consider: How likely is it that the hazard could harm me or someone else? How badly could I or someone else be harmed?

Ensure that you document and report any hazards that you are unable to deal with yourself, particularly if the hazard could cause serious harm to anyone. If necessary, seek instructions and training prior to using any equipment. If moving heavy loads, ask for help. Always adhere to local policy and procedure. If you think a work practice might be dangerous, this must be reported to your manager

Make the changes – The employer is responsible for attending to any hazards. Sometimes you may be able to fix simple hazards, but you must never put yourself or others at risk. You can tidy away any trailing cords or leads so as to eliminate a trip hazard. Getting rid of a hazard is the best way to fix it. In making hazards less dangerous, think about:

- Elimination (avoid any hazards by undertaking risk assessments).
- Substitution (are there any less hazardous ways of doing the task/procedure).
- Isolate/separate the hazard from people, by marking the area as a hazardous area.
- Safeguards (institute safeguards, for example, by knowing how to use equipment, the correct procedure to move heavy objects).
- Instructing others (enforce safe work procedures).
- Using personal protective equipment and clothing.

56 Clinical audit

At the point of registration, the Nursing Associate will be able to: participate in data collection to support audit activity, and contribute to the implementation of quality improvement strategies.

Figure 56.1   Stages of the audit cycle (Source: Redrawn from Healthcare Quality Improvement Partnership, 2020b).

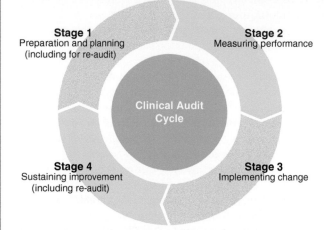

Stage 1
Preparation and planning
(including for re-audit)

Stage 2
Measuring performance

Clinical Audit Cycle

Stage 4
Sustaining improvement
(including re-audit)

Stage 3
Implementing change

Top Tip
Audit is an effective way of improving the quality of patient care by looking at current practice and modifying it where necessary.

Clinical audit is one way in which to find out if healthcare is being provided in line with set standards, and allows both those who provide care and patients to know where their service is doing well and where there could be improvements.

The overarching aim is to allow quality improvement to take place where it will be most beneficial and improve outcomes for patients. Clinical audit is one of a range of quality improvement methodologies that can deliver improved processes and outcomes for service users from a national perspective (national clinical audits) and audits performed locally in trusts, hospitals, GP practice, prisons and anywhere healthcare is provided. The focus in this chapter is on local audits.

Florence Nightingale

Florence Nightingale undertook one of the first clinical audits during the Crimean War. Shocked at the unsanitary conditions and the high mortality rates at Scutari, Nightingale and her nurses adopted stringent sanitary routines and standards of hygiene. Nightingale gathered data and kept records of mortality rates amongst patients. After the initiation of her sanitary and hygiene regime, mortality rates dropped from 40% to 2%. Her systemic approach is seen as one of the first programmes of outcomes management.

Audit

Clinical audit is not just a data collection exercise; it involves measuring current patient care and outcomes against explicit audit criteria (standards). From the outset, there is an expectation that practice will be improved. Clinical audit is defined as 'a quality improvement cycle that involves measurement of the effectiveness of healthcare against agreed and proven standards for high quality and taking action to bring practice in line with these standards so as to improve the quality of care and health outcomes'.

There are distinct statutory and contractual requirements for clinical audit that healthcare providers have to meet. The statutory and mandatory frameworks that regulate clinical audit within the NHS are continuing to evolve.

Stages of the audit cycle

Clinical audit is undertaken when there is a need for improvements to a service. The key is to ensure that re-audit is undertaken following implementation of changes made. There may be a need to undertake several re-audits so as to improve a service and sign off actions as complete (see Figure 56.1).

Stage one: preparation and planning

Good preparation is key to the success of an audit project. Identify available resources that will help in conducting the audit. Project management includes topic selection, planning, resources and communication. From the outset, project methodology, which includes design, data issues, implementation, involvement of stakeholders along with the provision of support for local improvement. The topic chosen should be a high priority for the organisation. This could involve areas in which there are high risks or high care costs (human and material), or an area that patients may have identified as a priority. Criteria must be decided on, and this is usually in the form of a statement. Recommendations from clinical practice guidelines such as National Institute for Health and Care Excellence (NICE) or Scottish Intercollegiate Guidelines Network (SIGN) can help to develop criteria and standards.

Stage two: measuring performance

An audit pro forma can be used for collecting data often derived from established guidelines and protocols. The data may be available in a computerised system, but it can also be collected manually depending on the outcome being measured, which can be retrospective or prospective. The data collected are then analysed, comparing the actual performance with the set standard.

Stage three: implementing change

There is little value in collecting data and little chance of making any impact unless it is followed with the implementation of change. The results should be presented and discussed with the relevant teams in the organisation and used to develop an action plan. The action plan describes recommendations and specifies what needs to be done, how it is to be done, who is going to do it and by when.

Stage four: sustaining improvement

This stage is key to the successful outcome of an audit. It follows up the previous stages of the audit, to ascertain whether the actions that have been taken have been effective, or if further improvements are needed. This involves repeating the audit cycle.

57 Risk assessment tools

At the point of registration, the Nursing Associate will be able to: accurately undertake risk assessments, using contemporary assessment tools.

Table 57.1 Some assessment tools.

Tool	Comment
Wound assessment tools	Several tools are available for the assessment of wounds. No tool has been identified which meets all the requirements of all practitioners.
Nutritional assessment tools	Malnutrition Universal Screening Tool (MUST) calculator is used in a number of care settings, establishing nutritional risk by using objective measurements (see Table 57.2).
National Early Warning Score (NEWS) 2	NEWS2 is established on a scoring system. A score is allocated to six physiological measurements that are already taken in hospitals, respiratory rate, oxygen saturations, temperature, systolic blood pressure, pulse rate and level of consciousness.
Abbreviated mental test (or AMT or mini-mental or MMSE)	Used to rapidly to assess patients for the possibility of dementia, delirium, confusion and other cognitive impairment.

Table 57.2 Components of Malnutrition Universal Screening Tool (British Association for Parenteral and Enteral Nutrition 2018).

Component	Description
BMI	Clinical impression – thin, acceptable weight, overweight. Clear wasting (very thin) and obesity (very overweight) may also be recorded.
Unplanned weight loss	Clothes and/or jewellery have become loose/fitting (weight loss), dentures may be loose. History of a decline in food intake, a reduction in appetite or swallowing problems over 3-6 months and underlying disease or psycho-social/physical disabilities that are likely to cause weight loss.
Acute disease and effect	Acutely ill as well as no nutritional intake or possibility of no intake for more than 5 days. If the patient is currently affected by an acute pathophysiological or psychological condition and there has been no nutritional intake or possibility of no intake for more than 5 days, it is likely that they will be at nutritional risk. These patients would include those who are critically ill, those who have swallowing difficulties (e.g. after stroke), or head injuries or those undergoing gastrointestinal surgery.

Determine overall risk of malnutrition
The result of the estimated BMI category, any unplanned weight loss and acute disease effect then allows the nurse to select the appropriate risk category.

Low	Medium	High

Top Tip

Any risk assessment tool is only there to support clinical judgement. The tool is only as good as the person who is using it. The significance of clinical judgement must never be underestimated.

The Nursing Associate at a Glance, First Edition. Ian Peate.
© 2021 John Wiley & Sons Ltd. Published 2021 by John Wiley & Sons Ltd.

ursing Associates contribute to most aspects of care, including delivery and monitoring; Registered Nurses will take the lead on assessment, planning and evaluation. The Nursing Associate must always work within their scope of practice and adhere to the tenets enshrined in the Code.

Providing care and support to people means the Nursing Associate has to use appropriate risk assessment tools to ascertain the ongoing need for support and intervention that people need. This requires the Nursing Associate to use appropriate assessment tools to determine, manage and escalate concerns.

Risk assessment tools

Nursing assessment requires the gathering of information regarding a patient's physiological, psychological, sociological and spiritual status. The appropriate use of assessment tools is to help the nurse to determine a balanced assessment that leads to a plan of care that meets the patient's individual needs.

Various patient risk assessments tools are available (Chapter 55 of this text discusses risk assessment tools in relation to health and safety). The various tools are intended to help nurses to provide safe and evidenced-based care. A list of the most popular nursing assessments tools used in practice includes everything from pain management to ensuring adequate staffing.

There is no instrument or tool used in clinical practice that is perfect. There are a number of reasons why a tool may have limitations: it can be a challenge to measure abstract concepts such as anxiety and pain, and errors may be caused by the instrument itself, the person using the tool, or how the tool is used with the population being assessed.

Risk prediction generally means using a systematic and proven method of identifying those who may be likely to deteriorate or suffer an exacerbation of a pre-existing risk. Risk management allows practitioners to minimise both the risk itself and the consequences of an adverse event. It can also provide an early-warning system maximising the probability of a positive outcome.

Tools and instruments

There are many names given to assessment tools. The name often reflects the purpose of the tool:

- Instruments
- Screening tools
- Screening instruments
- Risk assessment tools
- Risk assessment instruments
- Clinical algorithms

See Table 57.1 for an overview of assessment tools. Healthcare workers rely on tools or instruments to assist them when they assess a patient's health status and how the patient is progressing (outcomes). The various tools are used to help quantify and to objectively measure phenomena, for example, the size of a pressure sore; or to attempt to measure subjective concepts such as the level of anxiety. The use of an assessment tool helps to measure. The tools are used in conjunction with the assessment process and also as a part of an appraisal of risk. They may be handwritten or electronic. Risk assessment tools aim to predict the development of a patient's level of risk, for example, the risk that a patient will develop a pressure sore or that the patient's condition could change (for example, National Early Warning Score 2 (NEWS2) (see also Chapter 58)). When a risk has been identified, appropriate interventions must be put in place to mitigate the risk.

Those using and acting on scores derived from assessment tools should not rely solely on the scores, instruments and scales when assessing an individual. They must take into account other factors, for example, the degree of impairment, length of episode, history of the condition, family history, other co-morbid disorders and specific circumstances that are related to the patient.

Limitations

The instrument rating scale, an assessment tool, aims to objectify data that may be seen as subjective, for example, pain, anxiety and the size of a wound. Choosing the right tool and questioning its authority are important to ensure that the most appropriate tool is used and that safe, effective and patient-centred care is provided. All tools have potential limitations. To use any tool or instrument, the Nursing Associate needs to fully understand how to use the tool, apply it to clinical practice, act on the findings and document the action taken, if any. If no actions were taken after the assessment, the reason for this should be documented.

58 National Early Warning Score (NEWS2)

At the point of registration, the Nursing Associate will be able to: respond to and escalate potential hazards that may affect the safety of people.

Figure 58.1 NEWS2 physiological parameters (Source: RCP 2017).

Physiological parameter	Score						
	3	2	1	0	1	2	3
Respiration rate (per minute)	≤8		9–11	12–20		21–24	≥25
SpO₂ Scale 1 (%)	≤91	92–93	94–95	≥96			
SpO₂ Scale 2 (%)	≤83	84–85	86–87	88–92 ≥93 on air	93–94 on oxygen	95–96 on oxygen	≥97 on oxygen
Air or oxygen?		Oxygen		Air			
Systolic blood pressure (mmHg)	≤90	91–100	101–110	111–219			≥220
Pulse (per minute)	≤40		41–50	51–90	91–110	111–130	≥131
Consciousness				Alert			CVPU
Temperature (°C)	≤35.0		35.1–36.0	36.1–38.0	38.1–39.0	≥39.1	

Table 58.1 NEWS2 early warning scores and responses (Source: RCP, 2017).

NEWS2 Score	Frequency of monitoring	Clinical response
0	Minimum 12 hourly	Continue routine NEWS2 monitoring with each set of observations
Total: 1–4	Minimum 4–6 hourly	Inform Registered Nurse who must assess the patient Registered Nurse decides if increased frequency of monitoring and/or escalation of clinical care is needed
Total: 5 or more or 3 in one parameter	Increase frequency to a minimum of 1 hourly	Registered Nurse urgently informs medical team Urgent assessment by a clinician with competence to assess acutely ill patients Clinical care in an environment with monitoring facilities
Total: 7 or more	Continuous monitoring of vital signs	Registered Nurse immediately informs medical team at least at specialist registrar level Emergency assessment by a clinical team with critical care competence Consider transfer of clinical care to level 2 or 3 care facility

Top Tip

Failing to identify or act on signs that a patient's condition is deteriorating will result in a serious patient safety issue regardless of the care setting.

The Nursing Associate at a Glance, First Edition. Ian Peate.
© 2021 John Wiley & Sons Ltd. Published 2021 by John Wiley & Sons Ltd.

National Early Warning Scores (NEWS)

The use of early warning scores (EWS) was first introduced by the Department of Health in 2000, due in part to the recommendations made in the comprehensive critical care report. The EWS, also known as 'track-and-trigger systems', is the calculation of an aggregate trigger score based on physiological abnormalities. It is intended to provide support to objective decision-making so as to help healthcare staff identify deteriorating patients.

Failing to identify or act on signs that a patient's condition is deteriorating will result in a serious patient safety issue. It can mean that an opportunity may be missed to provide the essential care that could result in the best possible chance of survival. EWS can reliably detect deterioration in adults, triggering review and treatment as well as the escalation of care. When used appropriately, EWS such as NEWS2 can help the Nursing Associate to respond to and escalate potential hazards that could affect the safety of people.

In England, the National Institute for Health and Care Excellence (NICE) have recommended that adult patients in acute hospitals should have physiological observations recorded at initial assessment or on admission. Physiological observations should then be monitored at least every 12 hours, unless there has been a decision made at a senior level to increase or decrease the frequency of the monitoring for an individual patient. Physiological track-and-trigger systems should be used to monitor all adult patients in acute hospitals, with multiple-parameter or aggregated weighted scoring systems used to set trigger thresholds locally. NEWS2 is the track-and-trigger system recommended by NICE.

The Royal College of Physicians (RCP) have suggested that NEWS2 should be used when managing patients with COVID-19. The use of NEWS2 ensures that patients who are deteriorating, or at risk of deteriorating, will have a timely initial assessment undertaken by a competent clinical decision-maker. NEWS2 should always supplement clinical judgement in assessing a patient's condition.

National Early Warning Score 2

NEWS2 is a tool developed by the RCP which improves the detection and response to clinical deterioration in adult patients and is a key element of patient safety and improvement of patient outcomes. It is used across NHS England and in all ambulance trusts. In December 2017, a revised version was developed (NEWS2).

This early warning system has been shown to be an extremely effective system for the detection of patients who are at risk of clinical deterioration or death. The system when used correctly prompts a timely clinical response, aiming to improve patient outcomes. NEWS2 is a practical approach, with an emphasis on system-wide standardisation using physiological parameters that Nursing Associates and other staff are already measuring in hospitals. The findings of the assessment are recorded using a standardised clinical chart, the NEWS2 chart (see Figure 58.1).

NEWS2 uses a combined scoring system whereby a score is allocated to physiological measurements, with the magnitude of the score reflecting how extreme the variation from the norm is for the parameter, with a higher score representing further deviation from normal physiology and a higher risk of morbidity. A combined total is then arrived at, which is incremented by 2 points for those receiving additional oxygen required to maintain their recommended oxygen saturation. See Table 58.1 for scores and responses.

A holistic approach

Detection and management of patient deterioration are essential nursing competencies. Nursing Associates are expected to develop their observation, decision-making and communication skills in order to competently and confidently identify, interpret and respond to deterioration in a person's health. NEWS2 is used in England to support Nursing Associates in reducing adverse patient outcomes. Whilst NEWS2 is a useful tool for monitoring, recording and escalating vital signs, it must not be used in isolation; exploration of the wider clinical context is required in order to make safe and effective decisions.

59 Hazards and incidents

At the point of registration, the Nursing Associate will be able to: respond to and escalate potential hazards that may affect the safety of people.

Table 59.1 Some potential staff hazards.

Hazard	Description
Hazardous agents	These include biological agents (blood-borne pathogens), chemical agents, disinfectants and sterilants, antibiotics, hormones, chemotherapeutic agents, waste anaesthetic gases, latex gloves, aerosolised medications and hazardous waste.
Ergonomic hazards	These hazards include lifting, repetitive motion, standing for long periods of time and eye strain due to poor lighting.
Physical hazards	Physical hazards include toxic, reactive, corrosive or flammable compressed gases and chemicals; extreme temperatures that may cause burns or heat stress; mechanical hazards that could result in lacerations, punctures or abrasions; electrical hazards, radiation, noise, violence and slips and falls.
Psychological hazards	Psychological hazards are related to discrimination, technological changes, malfunctioning equipment, onerous work schedules, overwork, understaffing, excessive paperwork and bureaucracy, violence, dependent and demanding patients, patient deaths and lone working.

Table 59.2 Mistakes.

Adverse events	Action or failure to take action that then leads to unexpected, unintentional harm that could have been prevented.
Errors	Failure to do something the way it should have been done, for example, through bad planning or by being forgetful.
Near misses	Situations whereby an action might have harmed the person but did not, either by chance or purpose.
Incidents	Incidents are specific negative events. Serious incidents are described as events which need investigation as they caused severe harm or damage to either the person receiving care or to the organisation.

Top Tip

Whilst each event is unique, there are likely to be similarities and patterns in causes of risk that could otherwise go unnoticed if incidents are not reported and analysed.

Chapter 58 of this text has highlighted the need for the Nursing Associate to respond to and escalate any physiological changes that they may identify in a person's condition. Other potential hazards that may affect the safety of people exist, and it is equally important that these are also responded to and escalated appropriately.

Hazards to staff

The entire health and social care workforce are exposed them to a variety of hazards. For example, nursing staff are confronted with potential hazards such as exposure to infectious diseases and toxic substances, back injuries, radiation exposure and stress. Housekeeping staff (for example, cleaners) can be exposed to cleaning materials and disinfectants that can result in rashes and eye and throat irritation and to infectious diseases. Maintenance workers may have to confront electrical, asbestos and solvent hazards.

Despite this diversity of occupations and exposures, healthcare hazards can be divided into four categories: hazardous agents, ergonomic hazards, physical hazards and psychological hazards (see Table 59.1). Awareness of the hazards in Table 59.1 and implementation of appropriate precautions may help to prevent injuries and illnesses to staff. Any threat to health and safety must be reported to the appropriate person so that action can be taken (see also Chapter 57).

Incidents, error and near misses

Despite adhering to the best ways of working, there will always be potential risks that could lead to patient harm. The Nursing Associate and other team members must work in a collaborative manner towards the well-being of those who require care or support. Mistakes can happen as a result of one of the following:

- Lack of knowledge and understanding
- Poor communication
- Failure to share information
- Stress
- Negligence
- Failure to pay attention (being distracted)

The Nursing Associate has a duty to ensure that adverse events, incidents, errors and near misses have been documented and reported accurately. To do this effectively, there is a need to be able to understand them so that they can be recognised.

Mistakes can occur due to adverse events, errors and near misses (see Table 59.2).

Patient safety reporting systems

The most important knowledge in the field of patient safety is how to prevent harm to people as they receive treatment and care. One of the most basic functions of patient safety reporting systems is to improve safety by learning from the failures of the healthcare system. Healthcare errors are usually triggered by weak systems and often have common root causes, which can often be generalised and corrected. Whilst each event is unique, there are likely to be similarities and patterns in causes of risk that could otherwise go unnoticed if incidents are not reported and analysed.

A reporting system would generally have the following components:

Description (what happened): Patient characteristics (such as age, gender); incident characteristics (observations, measurements, clinical features, tentative disease categories); the location (hospital, clinic,); people involved; how, when and by whom the incident was noticed; the possible harm (direct and consequential) and immediate action taken to remedy the situation.

Explanation (why it happened): A set of known risks associated with the patient's condition, causes of the event, contributing factors or mitigating factors.

Remedial measures (what were the reactions): For example, the identification of weak links in the care chain, review of clinical and supervisory processes and procedures, as well as administrative, educational and other requirements to prevent a repetition of similar incidents to minimise impact on the patient and on the care organisation if it occurs again.

Escalating concerns

Immediately after an adverse event, incident, error or near miss occurs, ensure that the needs of the individuals involved are addressed. This may require the application of first aid or calling emergency services, or it may suffice to chat with the person to determine that they are fine. The Nursing Associate should inform their manager next and adhere to local policy and procedure at all times. Patient safety reporting systems are varied; reporting is an important step for improving patient safety. Complete the relevant paperwork; often this is known as an incident form or accident form, or it may be an electronic system.

60 Staffing and safe care

At the point of registration, the Nursing Associate will be able to: recognise when inadequate staffing levels impact the ability to provide safe care and escalate concerns appropriately.

Table 60.1 The Code and safe staffing levels.

Issue	What the Code says
Environmental factors such as staffing levels can affect the Nursing Associates' ability to uphold the values of the Code.	The Nursing Associate must put the interests of people using or needing their services first. The Nursing Associate must make the care and safety of people their main concern and ensure that their dignity is preserved.
Putting the interests of people first, the primary duty means that the Nursing Associate should be vigilant about safety and quality.	The Nursing Associate must work with colleagues to evaluate the quality of their work and that of the team. The Nursing Associate must work with colleagues to preserve the safety of those receiving care.
The Nursing Associate has a professional duty to act or speak out if quality and safety could be compromised.	The Nursing Associate must act without delay if they believe that there is a risk to patient safety or public protection. The Nursing Associate must raise and, if necessary, escalate any concerns that they may have about patient or public safety, or the level of care people are receiving in the workplace or any other healthcare setting, and use the channels available to them in line with Nursing and Midwifery Council (NMC) guidance and local working practices.
The NMC require Nursing Associates to uphold existing legislation and nationally agreed standards as well as the Code.	The Nursing Associate must tell someone in authority at the first reasonable opportunity if they are experiencing problems that could prevent them working within the Code or other national standards.

Box 60.1 Primary responsibilities of the Nursing Associate.

- Communicating, maintaining and monitoring standards
- Ensuring the correct number of staff equipped with the necessary knowledge and skills
- Ensuring the appropriate resources
- Ensuring the environment is safe and fit for purpose
- Asking for advice and support when necessary

Box 60.2 Steps to be taken in raising concerns.

Prior to thinking about raising a concern, consider these questions:

- Have I done anything to try to address the situation within my own resources?
- Are there any other options available to me?
- Is there anything more that I can do prior to involving my manager?
- Could I prioritise things to reduce the impact on the patient?
- What is my specific concern?
- What do I need to help me deal with this situation safely?
- What is it that I want from my manager?

When these options have been considered and you have done what you can to address the immediate situation, decide what the next appropriate course of action should be. Normally, concerns should be raised internally with the line manager in the first instance, either verbally or in writing. Keep a record of the concern raised. Concerns can be raised by e-mail or letter and/or by using the incident-reporting system. If you feel unable to raise your concern with the line manager, raise your concern with the designated person in your organisation.

Top Tip

The work of the Nursing Associate is complex and cognitively and managerially demanding, Appropriate staffing levels are essential.

The Nursing Associate at a Glance, First Edition. Ian Peate.
© 2021 John Wiley & Sons Ltd. Published 2021 by John Wiley & Sons Ltd.

Chapter 59 has identified some of the hazards and incidents that may put the safety of patients and staff at risk. This chapter considers inadequate staffing levels and the impact that this may have on the Nursing Associate's ability to offer safe care. Reduced or inadequate staffing levels can also impact the health and well-being of staff.

Skill mix

There is a great deal of variation in what is meant by skill mix (sometimes referred to as personnel mix). Skill mix can mean the mix of posts within the establishment; the mix of employees in a post; the combination of skills that are available at a particular time; or it could refer to the combinations of activities comprising each role, as opposed to the combination of different job titles. The skill mix includes the skills and experience of staff, their continuing professional development, years of experience and how they combine these to form their professional judgement.

Shortages of nurses have been linked to poor care in hospitals. It is challenging for researchers to be specific as to the number and type of staff needed, or to be certain that staffing levels are indeed the root of the problem. It is acknowledged that increased staffing levels cost more, and as such there are financial perspectives to be taken into consideration.

An increasing body of evidence demonstrates how appropriate nurse staffing leads to improved patient outcomes. In hospitals, researchers have determined that those patients who spent time on wards with fewer than the usual number of Registered Nurses caring for them were more likely to die or stay in hospital for longer periods. When staffing levels were lower, more observations (vital signs such as, blood pressure and pulse) were missed, and this was associated with higher death rates. However, low staffing could not explain why most of the observations were being missed. Levels of healthcare assistants were also found to be important, and deaths could be reduced at the lowest cost by replacing some healthcare assistants with Registered Nurses. Caution needs to be exercised as the research design meant that there could be no certainty regarding cause and effect.

In the hospital setting, the nursing staff usually represent the largest single occupational group. As a result of this, efforts to manage hospital costs can often involve cutting nursing care, reducing the number of nurses or replacing professional nursing staff with other staff such as assistive personnel.

Impact of inadequate staffing levels

The heavy workload of nurses is a major problem within health and social care settings, it has many manifestations, including fatigue, and it lowers morale amongst staff, which is a threat to patient safety. Nurses are experiencing higher workloads than ever before due to an increased demand for nurses coupled with an inadequate supply of nurses, reduced staffing and a reduction in patient length of stay.

The primary responsibility of the Nursing Associate is to ensure that patients within their area of clinical responsibility receive care that is safe and effective. This is achieved in a number of ways (see Box 60.1).

The Nursing and Midwifery Council

The NMC acknowledge that appropriate staffing has an important part to play in the delivery of safe and effective healthcare. Safe staffing, they declare, must be matched to the individual patients' needs and concerns skill mix as well as numbers, is about other staff as well as nurses and applies to other settings as well as to hospitals. Setting or assuring standards related to appropriate staffing is not the job of the NMC, yet it has an impact on how the NMC undertake professional regulation.

The Code provides the core standards of ethics and practice that are expected from registrants, and this means all registrants, including senior managers. See Table 60.1 for what the Code expects of registrants in relation to staffing. These statements are intended to support registrants so they can ensure that their practice meets the standard required of the professions.

If the Nursing Associate feels that their ability to ensure delivery of safe and effective care is being compromised, their duty is to communicate these concerns to their line manager using locally agreed policies and procedures (see Box 60.2). Making their line manager aware of the situation gives them an opportunity to resolve the issue or escalate the concerns to the next level.

61 Revalidation

At the point of registration, the Nursing Associate will be able to: understand the need for revalidation and the requirements made by the Nursing and Midwifery Council (NMC).

Figure 61.1   Some aspects of revalidation (NMC 2018a and b).

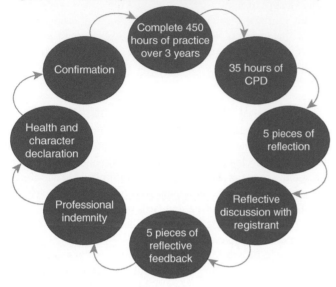

Box 61.1   The revalidation process.

- An online account is required
- A portfolio should be created – these can be self-made or commercially purchased
- A log of practice hours (350 hours)
- A record of continuing professional development – 35 hours with a minimum of 20 hours participatory
- Feedback on practice (five examples are required)
- Five written reflections
- Undertake a reflective discussion with another registrant
- Confirmation
- Submission

Top Tip

Revalidation emphasises the professional development of those who are on the register, which can be used to support the conditions in which better, safer care can flourish.

Whilst the important issue of revalidation is not a requirement of the Standards of Proficiency for Nursing Associates, it is an important aspect that deserves its own chapter.

In January 2019, the Nursing and Midwifery Council (NMC) began to accept individuals onto the Nursing Associate part of the register. It is an offence for anyone to practise or claim to be a Nursing Associate in England without being qualified and registered. Nursing Associates are required to register and continue to meet the standards laid out in the Code as a condition of their registration. The NMC regulate Nursing Associates in broadly the same way that they regulate Nurses and Midwives, which includes registration, revalidation and fitness to practise. The Nursing Associate pays the same registration fees as Nurses and Midwives, and every three years their registration will need to be renewed through the same revalidation process applicable to Nurses and Midwives.

Revalidation

Revalidation is the method by which the Nursing Associate renews their registration. The purpose of revalidation is to enhance public protection by ensuring the Nursing Associate remains fit to practise throughout their career. Revalidation reinforces your duty to maintain your fitness to practise within your own scope of practice, encouraging you to incorporate the Code as you practise day in day out and as a part of your personal development. Revalidation encourages engagement in professional networks and discussions. It also has the potential to reduce professional isolation. Employer engagement is also enhanced with revalidation, increasing access and participation in appraisals and continuing professional development. Revalidation involves the collection and storage of evidence to demonstrate that the Nursing Associate can practise safely and effectively. Revalidation replaces the previous post registration education and practice (PREP) system by introducing eight core components (see Figure 61.1).

The Nursing Associate's responsibility

The Nursing Associate is responsible for their own revalidation application. Planning ahead is essential to ensure, to the best of their ability, that they will meet the requirements within their three-year renewal period. It is expected that revalidation is completed online, and it must never be delegated to another person unless the NMC have given their permission for an adjustment. The information that is provided in the online application must be accurate. A step-by-step approach to revalidation is shown in Box 61.1.

The NMC acknowledge that there may be circumstances that make it more difficult for some registrants to meet the revalidation requirements. For example, if the registrant has a disability, is ill, pregnant, a maternity period or if another life event impacts the person's ability to meet the revalidation requirements. They may permit an extension to the revalidation date (extensions cannot be longer than six weeks) or provide assistance with the online application. Prepare for revalidation by:

- Joining the NMC online and knowing when your renewal date is
- Ensuring that the NMC has your most up-to-date contact details
- Becoming familiar with the Code
- Reading the NMC guidance regarding revalidation
- Ensuring that revalidation, from the moment you register, is in your mind, particularly Continuing Professional Development (CPD) hours
- Using your annual appraisal, if appropriate, for your revalidation preparation and confirmation

Practice-related feedback

Nursing Associates are required to obtain and provide the NMC with five pieces of reflective feedback in the three-year period since their registration was last renewed or they joined the register.

Nursing Associates already receive a range of feedback, and the five pieces of feedback collected for revalidation can come from a variety of sources and in a number of forms. The feedback can be written or verbal, formal or informal, from patients, teachers, researchers, colleagues and management. It could also include feedback from team performance reports, the annual appraisal or clinical supervision. Keep a note of the content of any feedback received, and include how you used it to improve your practice. What is important is that you do not record any information which may identify another person (patients or staff).

Written reflection

Nursing Associate are required to have prepared five written reflective accounts in the three-year period since their registration was last renewed or they joined the register. The reflective account must be recorded on the approved form and must refer to an instance of their CPD, a piece of practice-related feedback, an event or experience in practice or a combination of all three. They must all relate to the Code.

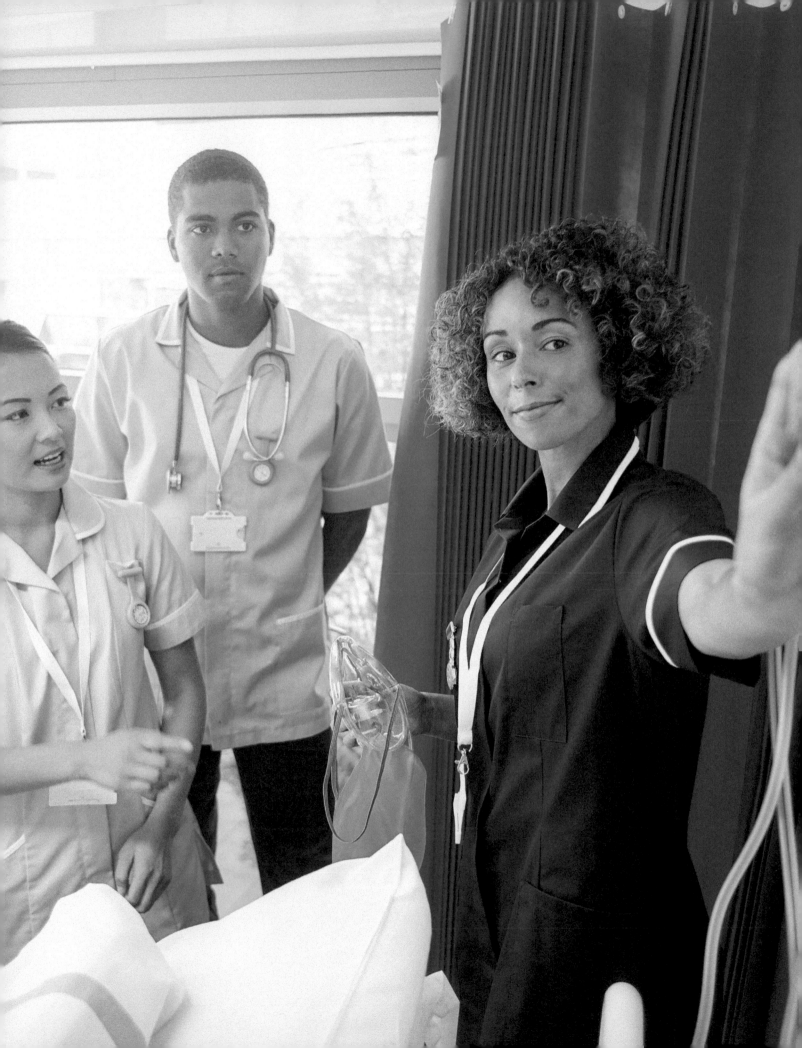

Contributing to integrated care

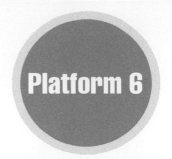

62 Being resilient

At the point of registration, the Nursing Associate will be able to: recognise uncertainty and demonstrate an awareness of strategies to develop resilience in themselves, know how to seek support to help deal with uncertain situations.

Box 62.1   Seven key areas associated with being resilient (Source: Adapted RCN, 2016).

1 Attending to and taking care of your basic needs
2 Enjoying emotional stability
3 Being confident
4 Having social support systems available
5 Speaking your truth
6 Seeking insight and self-awareness
7 Having faith

Box 62.2   How resilient am I?

There are a number of tests available online to help you identify how resilient you are.
　Search online to find many more examples of inventories and guides to assessing and improving your resilience.
　This quick test may help you in taking stock: www.resiliencyquiz.com
　This is another free online test: www.testyourrq.com

Top Tip
Resilient individuals are recognised by their confidence (self-efficacy), coordination (planning), control, composure (low anxiety), commitment (persistence) as well as by their ability to make adversity meaningful.

Resilience

Resilience has been explained as the ability to succeed, to live and to develop in a positive way, in the face of stress or adversity that would usually involve the real possibility of a negative outcome. It is the ability to maintain personal well-being whilst working in the face of challenge. One of the greatest challenges the NHS faces is workforce resilience, capacity and well-being.

Resilience allows the Nursing Associate to withstand setbacks, deal with frustrations and manage personal tragedies. During a crisis (for example, the COVID-19 pandemic), the person who demonstrates their ability to be resilient will do their best to cope with events and incidents in a calm manner, with patience, acceptance and also hope. Those who are less resilient could respond with anger, fear and dread, frustration and impatience and see themselves as the victim. There are seven key areas that can help make a person resilient (see Box 62.1). Maslow proposed a hierarchy of human needs, which is usually represented as a pyramid, where it was necessary for one need to be fulfilled so as to meet the next. The lower needs, such as food and shelter, air and water need to be met so as to move on to attaining the next level of needs. With regard to resilience, those seven key areas associated with needs (Box 62.1) can also be considered as a hierarchy. The Nursing Associate has to attain each one to develop and sustain resilience.

Being a resilient Nursing Associate is an important quality to have. Caring for people in a variety of care settings and often with complex physical, mental, emotional needs can be demanding. This can often challenge staff, impacting their own health and well-being negatively, and the outcome can be detrimental to their performance. See Box 62.2.

Basic needs

Attending to and taking care of your basic needs requires the Nursing Associate to look after themselves, their health and to ensure that they are eating a balanced diet and sleeping well. They need to respond to what the body needs, what is required to promote rest, keep well and remain physically and psychologically strong. Exercising and taking regular breaks can help to recharge energy levels and enhance mood.

Emotional stability

Sometimes, caring for people and their families can cause uncomfortable and difficult emotions. Being able to adjust your emotional response to demonstrate emotional stability and predictability is essential for dealing with challenging situations. Reflection, breathing techniques, meditation and mindfulness are suggested approaches to inducing and maintaining calm. You should, if appropriate, attend clinical supervision sessions to help you with emotional stability.

Confidence

Being confident, having positive self-esteem, as well as a belief in your capacity to address and deal with negative setbacks is at the heart of being resilient. Working within a team requires cooperation between team members, and doing your part is critical to providing the best possible care. It is important to believe in yourself and the care that you are delivering.

Social support

Effective relationships and support networks are essential for handling any difficult situations. Make use of people who want to help you. This could be a colleague or a friend when you feel your workload is getting too much. You cannot do everything, and nobody should expect you to. Over-engagement with work (not having a work life balance) can have negative consequences, and lead to health and well-being problems for you and those at home. Make your home a sanctuary and connect with people. Invest in personal relationships.

Speaking your truth (be honest with yourself)

Caring for a person can bring your own mortality into focus. You might want to talk about this. Feeling this way and acknowledging this is OK, and talking about it can help you. Being honest about your fears, vulnerability and needs is essential as you work through challenging situations.

Self-awareness and insight

Having an understanding and being aware of what has led to a challenging situation can help change behaviour. You may reflect and conclude that you did not manage a particular situation well, or perhaps a patient or a member of their family became angry for some reason.

Having faith

Faith is not just about believing in a higher being or being spiritual; it is about believing in life and trusting yourself. Difficult situations may bring a crisis of faith. Faith can also mean acting empathically, forgiving and having compassion and appreciation.

63 The roles of health and social care teams

At the point of registration, the Nursing Associate will be able to: understand their own role and the roles of all other staff at different levels of experience and seniority in the event of a major incident.

Figure 63.1 The four key factors.

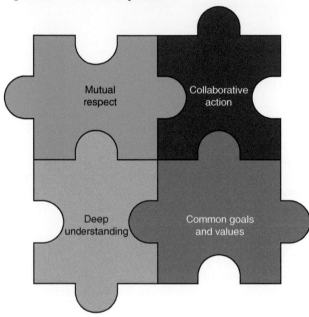

Mutual respect

Collaborative action

Deep understanding

Common goals and values

Top Tip

A major incident is any emergency requiring the implementation of special arrangements by one or all of the emergency services and will generally include the involvement of large numbers of people.

A team is a small number of people who have complementary skills, who are committed to a common purpose and have set performance goals for which they hold each other jointly accountable. An effective team is dependent upon how well its members work together to achieve shared goals.

No health and social care member of staff should ever practise in isolation. Working in a collaborative manner is an essential component of a highly functioning and effective health and care service. Whilst individual organisations and agencies may have specific responsibilities during a major incident , there must also be a combined and coordinated response. Teams bring together the skills, experiences and disciplines required to support people.

Adopting a collaborative approach can improve communication, save time, reduce duplication of work, improve working relationships and provide a better experience for people who use health and social care services.

Integrated care

Integrated care is also known as integrated health, coordinated care, comprehensive care, seamless care or transmural care. It focuses on more coordinated and integrated forms of care provision. It is care that is planned with people working together to understand the service user and their carer(s). The aim is to put them in control. Integrated care coordinates and delivers services so as to achieve the best outcomes. Integrated care aims to improve the patient experience, accomplish higher levels of efficiency and enhance value from health delivery systems and address fragmentation in patient services, enabling more coordinated and continuous care.

Integrated care in the NHS is a term that is generally used to mean either more joined-up services, such as community care teams involving health and social care professionals and more closely linked organisations, for example, NHS organisations working with one another, or NHS organisations working with non-NHS organisations.

Effective working relationships

Effective working relationships are essential in generating energy and ideas for improvements. Team relationships are complex, and there is a need to know how well members of the team work together, to engender good working relationships and to identify how improvements can be made.

If relationships between the teams are poor, this should be acknowledged from the outset. If the relationship is already good, the team members can work together to decide how the team can work even better. One important aim is to ensure that interactions between team members create energy and to think of new and innovative ideas so as to improve care and thus patient outcomes.

There are four key factors that are often referred to as key to helping change, fitting together as if part of a jigsaw puzzle (see Figure 63.1):

1 Mutual respect for each other's unique role, identifying potential for contribution and expertise
2 Deep understanding of each other; this happens best by active conversation
3 Collaborative action where team members work together, make mistakes together and learn together
4 Common goals and values that go beyond differences in the team

Understanding roles

Adopting an integrated approach can enable workers to understand each other's roles and contributions as well as building support networks around individuals. Integrated working will affect people's roles and professional identities. Health and care workers can maintain their sense of professional identity and at the same time work across boundaries that are becoming more and more blurred. To achieve this, roles, responsibilities and accountability must be clearly described, this is so very important when a major incident has been declared. It is essential that local and national policies are made available and are understood so the response to a disaster or major incident can be effective.

If a team is to perform effectively, it is critical that all team members have a clear understanding of the various roles within the integrated team and that any misconceptions or myths concerning roles are dispelled. Failure to understand each other's roles and responsibilities has real potential to create tension, miscommunication, mistrust and inefficiency within the team. Generating a greater understanding of the various roles and constraints is an important foundation in building a more integrated team. Discussions about roles and constraints can help dispel myths and develop deeper insights and also enhance good levels of reciprocal understanding.

64 Long-term conditions

At the point of registration, the Nursing Associate will be able to: understand and explore the challenges of providing safe nursing care for people with complex co-morbidities and complex care needs.

Box 64.1   Long-term health conditions and mental health problems (Source: Naylor et al., 2012).

- Depression is two to three times more common in a range of cardiovascular diseases including cardiac disease, coronary artery disease, stroke, angina, congestive heart failure or following a heart attack
- People living with diabetes are two to three times more likely to have depression than the general population
- Mental health problems are around three times more prevalent among people with chronic obstructive pulmonary disease than in the general population; anxiety disorders are particularly common, for example, panic disorder
- Depression is common in people with chronic musculoskeletal disorders

Figure 64.1   The pyramid of care.

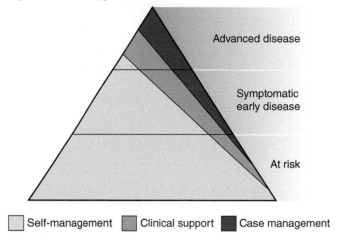

Advanced disease

Symptomatic early disease

At risk

☐ Self-management   ☐ Clinical support   ■ Case management

Top Tip

The scale of long-term conditions is a challenge for contemporary healthcare systems, a model of care which takes into account and acknowledges that the expertise and resources of people with long-term conditions and their communities is the way forward.

The Nursing Associate at a Glance, First Edition. Ian Peate.
© 2021 John Wiley & Sons Ltd. Published 2021 by John Wiley & Sons Ltd.

Long-term conditions or chronic diseases are conditions for which currently there is no cure. These conditions are managed with drugs and other treatment, and include asthma, epilepsy, diabetes, chronic obstructive pulmonary disease, arthritis and hypertension. People with long-term conditions are also more likely to experience mental health problems than the general population (see Box 64.1). People with long-term conditions and co-morbid mental health problems often live in deprived areas and disproportionately have access to fewer resources. When co-morbidities and deprivation come together, significant inequalities are generated and maintained.

Long-term conditions

The ongoing prevalence of long-term conditions is one of the biggest challenges that the NHS is facing. The NHS, social care and the voluntary sector are all working together to develop innovative and appropriate ways to reduce the burden of long-term conditions for individuals, communities and nations. There is a need to ensure that people are put at the centre of decisions that are being made about their care along with a focus on innovation that also embraces new technologies. The need to change organisational culture is essential so as to make a difference to the lives of people with long-term conditions.

People who are affected, or potentially affected, by long-term conditions have individual and differing complex needs. Those with long-term conditions can be intensive users of health and social care services, which includes community services, urgent and emergency care and acute services. Services have to be improved, and in so doing this can also improve efficiency. Preventive, personalised, integrated and innovative approaches to care provision have to become the norm in order to transform people's lives and achieve better quality and productivity.

The prevalence of long-term conditions is linked to age and socio-economic status. There are a number of other associated linked factors. Understanding the make-up and needs of the local population or community is vital to ensuring that care is suited to meet their needs, better supporting people to self-care and look after themselves, with patients in control of their conditions.

Personalised care planning

Personalised care planning is about involving people in decisions about their care, providing them with access to all of the information that they need to assist them as they make those decisions – 'no decision about me without me'.

Empowering patients to maximise self-management, shared decision-making and choice are key components of self-care for those with a long-term condition. This includes ensuring that patients are offered a care plan and the patient and those caring for them have access to the appropriate information about managing their condition. A systematic transfer of knowledge to patients is required for this to happen. It should be remembered that the best resources are the patients themselves. If patients are provided with support by health and social care professionals to have the confidence to take control and manage their conditions better, disease progression can be slowed and reliance on services reduced.

The pyramid of care for those with long-term conditions

The pyramid of care models long-term conditions by dividing the population into people who can care for themselves, those who need help to manage their conditions and those who need more intensive case management. Attempting to put populations into these groups is a complex activity. This is because of limited information, people moving between levels of the pyramid (see Figure 64.1) and the ways that different models of care can influence assessment of an individual's needs and where they are located in the pyramid. The majority of those with a long-term condition self-manage their own condition. This group may require the Nursing Associate or other health and care professionals to offer advice on health promotion. Another group comprises those with disease-specific unstable long-term conditions, and it is community nurses who are most likely to be involved in care provision. The final group are those with highly complex multiple conditions, requiring intense case management. Usually these people are cared for by a community matron or a case management worker. There are people with long-term conditions who can and do self-manage a number of complex medical regimens every day. This includes taking medicines, self-injecting therapies, dressing wounds and also dealing with the challenges that everyday living brings.

65 Promoting independence

At the point of registration, the Nursing Associate will be able to: understand the principles and processes involved in supporting people and families with a range of care needs to maintain optimal independence and avoid unnecessary interventions and disruptions to their lives.

Figure 65.1   Personalised goals.

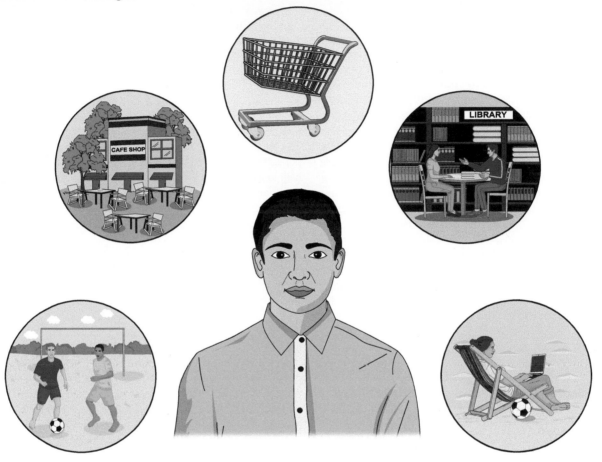

Box 65.1   Points to be considered when offering people support as they regain their confidence and independence.

- The person's wishes and quality of life
- Risks that are related to specific activities or the environment
- Think about actions that might help reduce any risk, for example, the use of equipment, reminders, the provision of support from others
- What effect taking the risk might have for the person as well as those staff who are supporting them.

Top Tip

During the decision-making process, consideration should be given to the risk of harm balanced against a person's right to freedom of action.

The Nursing Associate at a Glance, First Edition. Ian Peate.
© 2021 John Wiley & Sons Ltd. Published 2021 by John Wiley & Sons Ltd.

Intermediate care

Intermediate care requires health and social care professionals and organisations to work closely with people and agree what intensive support they need in order to improve their independence. Intermediate care is a short-term service that works towards specific goals. It is different from care and support that is ongoing. It is a multidisciplinary service offering support and rehabilitation to those whose condition has stabilised, enabling their transfer from hospital to the community or avoiding unnecessary admissions or readmissions.

Most of the patients affected by delayed transfers are those who are waiting for appropriate packages of care to allow them to be discharged. Delayed discharge puts patients at risk of infections, depression, loss of independence and confidence. It is also an inappropriate use of NHS resources. Increasingly, commissioning groups, local authorities and independent care providers are working together to provide intermediate care solutions that could alleviate the problem.

Core principles

The principles of care required to offer an intermediate service, and as such promote independence, include:

- Building an equal partnership – determine what it is that motivates the person and what they seek to achieve.
- Focusing on strengths – what can the person already do, and how can this be built upon?
- Building resilience and confidence – what might help the person feel more confident to manage daily living?
- Observing and encouraging – even when the person is finding an activity challenging, hold back if safe to do so and encourage them.
- Supporting positive risk-taking – consider the benefits of taking risks as well as the drawbacks of avoiding them.

Risk

It is important to encourage choice and control for people who require care and support. They should be assisted to do as much for themselves as possible. Each person is different, and some-times, for some, what may be seen as a simple task, such as being able to shave or to make a cup of tea for themselves, can be of great importance. Where there is potential or actual risk to health or safety, the Nursing Associate has to think of ways that the person can be supported so as to maintain their independence, as opposed to preventing them from doing those things that they want to do for themselves.

Offering support to people as they regain their confidence and independence will require some positive risk-taking. Risk assessment and planning can help to manage risk and to enhance an individual's potential for achieving their goals. Points to think about are discussed in Box 65.1.

Personalised goals

When promoting independence, it is important to choose the right goals. Agree goals with the person, taking into account what it is that is important to them and what it is that the service aims to achieve. Goals can involve things like taking part in social, leisure, sports activities, as well as practical or everyday tasks (see Figure 65.1). Ensure that the goals:

- Reflect the person's best interests and aspirations
- Can be measured
- Take into account the person's health and well-being
- Are what the person wants to achieve
- Consider how the individual's condition(s) or experiences affect them

Intermediate care and re-ablement services are crucial elements of national healthcare policy that can provide health and care closer to home and avoid hospital admissions or readmissions.

Greater integration across all aspects of the health and care system can help to slow the increase in hospitalisations and also improve the quality and experience of people's care. Intermediate care is at the forefront of NHS England's Five Year Forward View and Next Steps for the Five Year Forward View. It emphasises the need to help frail and older people stay healthy and independent, a key function of intermediate care.

A number of different professionals can deliver integrated care, from nurses and therapists to social workers. The person or the team providing the care plan must take into account the individual's needs at that time.

66 Accessing care

At the point of registration, the Nursing Associate will be able to: identify when people need help to facilitate equitable access to care, support, and escalate concerns appropriately.

Table 66.1 Barriers to accessing services.

Physical barriers	Objects that prevent an individual from getting where they want to get to (independently or otherwise), the lack of wheelchair access to a building, steps that prevent some patients from entering a building, absence of car parking for disabled people, narrow doors that cannot accommodate a wheelchair or other mobility device.
Psychological barriers	This barrier can impact the way a person thinks about a service. For example, they may have a fear of needles, or the service may be seen as stigmatising (for example, sexual health services). If an individual is unwell and is apprehensive about what is wrong with them, they may not seek help from their healthcare provider.
Financial barriers	The cost of accessing a service could be a barrier. Transport costs in getting to a service or having to pay for medical prescriptions could result in a person not getting the medicine or care that they need.
Geographical barriers	Whilst some individuals may live close to health and social care services, others may live some distance away. Having to get a bus or other form of transport may deter a person from accessing a service. This can be exacerbated if the person has a disability, and the transportation service fails to address their accessibility needs. A patient may require specialist treatment which is some distance away from their home, and they may find it a challenge to get there. The distance is a geographical barrier. Some people, due to their health or care needs, may be unable to mobilise and may not be able to walk a short distance to the health and social care service.
Cultural and language barriers	If information provided concerning health and social care services (signs, leaflets, posters) is in English only, those with a different first language may not be able to find out about services. If the information uses specialist language or jargon, the individual may not understand it, causing anxiety and worry. There may be a need to use British Sign Language or other forms of communication.
Resource barriers	Barriers also include lack of human (staff) and material resources (equipment and funding). If there is an excess demand for a service, people may have to wait for it.

Top Tip

The NHS is under a legal and moral obligation to provide services to all people who need them, regardless of their gender, age or ethnic background.

The Nursing Associate at a Glance, First Edition. Ian Peate.
© 2021 John Wiley & Sons Ltd. Published 2021 by John Wiley & Sons Ltd.

In the UK, since 1948 the NHS has provided universal, comprehensive healthcare that is free at the point of delivery. NHS services are provided based on clinical need and not on an individual's ability to pay. NHS services are free of charge, except in limited circumstances.

Despite this, there are inequities in healthcare in the UK, along with poorer access and worse patient outcomes that are strongly associated with social disadvantage.

The NHS England

The NHS is funded mainly through general taxation that is supplemented by National Insurance contributions. Whilst the NHS is often portrayed as being 'free at the point of use', since 1951 those using the service have been required to pay an additional contribution towards the cost of certain services, such as prescriptions and dental treatment. There are exception arrangements in place appropriate to many patients, including those aged under 16 or those 60 years and over, as well as those people who are in receipt of specific state benefits. Across the UK, private health insurance policies are held by some people. Often these are corporate subscriptions that are offered to employees as part of their overall salary package.

Access to services

People have the right to access NHS services, and they will not be refused access on unreasonable grounds. People will receive care and treatment that is appropriate to them and that meets their needs and reflects their preferences.

The NHS Constitution make clear that the NHS is required to assess the health requirements of communities and to commission and put in place the services required to meet those needs as considered necessary. In the case of public health services that have been commissioned by local authorities, it must take steps to improve the health of the local population. People have the right not to be unlawfully discriminated against in the provision of NHS services including on the grounds of gender, race, disability, age, sexual orientation, religion, belief, gender reassignment, pregnancy and maternity or marital or civil partnership status. Access to healthcare is an important principle that underpins the NHS philosophy; it is its driving aim. There are concerns, however, that some vulnerable groups (for example, socio-economically

disadvantaged people, people from a black and minority ethnic backgrounds) face greater difficulties in accessing healthcare than others. A range of factors can influence access to healthcare, particularly for vulnerable groups. People may be disadvantaged when they seek access to services because they may present late, can have difficulty in getting their concerns across or they could have problems such as obesity and smoking that may make them unsuitable for some forms of care. It could also be that there is not enough capacity in the system in order to meet everyone's needs. Access to healthcare is a difficult entity to measure accurately. It is dynamic and subject to change because of the characteristics of the service being offered, the patient attempting (or not) to access the service and how these interact. It is not as easy as simply looking at the number of appointments in the system and determining how many people attend and do not attend; it is far more complicated than this.

All those who access healthcare services have vulnerabilities when it comes to access. However, these vulnerabilities can be amplified if the person has less income or as a result of their ethnicity, age, gender and ability.

Barriers to accessing services

These are the factors that prevent a person from accessing health and social care services. Individuals can often face more than one barrier when trying to access services (see Table 66.1). Effective support can enable those seeking access to services to find the information that they need, access services and become more confident in advocating for themselves and their families.

Improving access to services

Improving access to services for vulnerable people is important if health equity is to be achieved. When the Nursing Associate understands the challenges that people may face, they may be more confident in assisting people when they need to use services. Innovative approaches are required to improve access for vulnerable populations and to determine which components of health systems, organisations or services are problematic, with the intention of making changes that can transform service provision.

Involving service users and people with lived experience in decision-making and service developments is essential so that services are responsive and relevant to local needs.

67 Discharge planning

At the point of registration, the Nursing Associate will be able to: demonstrate an understanding of their own role and contribution when involved in the care of a person who is undergoing discharge or a transition of care between professionals, settings or services.

Figure 67.1   People and services that may be a part of the discharge process.

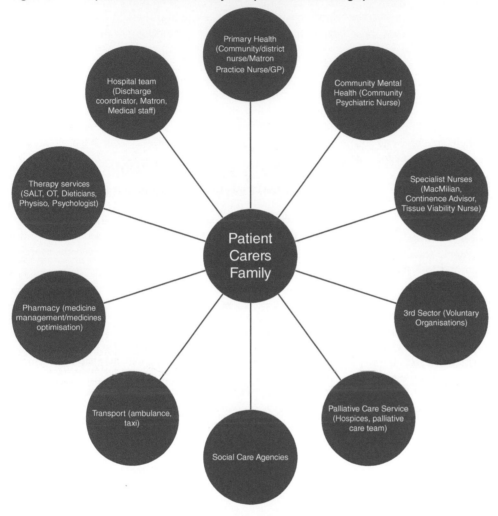

Top Tip

Safe, reliable healthcare is dependent on access to, and the use of, information that is accurate, valid, reliable, timely, relevant, legible and complete, and this equally applies to discharge.

The Nursing Associate at a Glance, First Edition. Ian Peate.
© 2021 John Wiley & Sons Ltd. Published 2021 by John Wiley & Sons Ltd.

Risks to patient safety can occur when they are discharged from hospital. Vital information may not have been transferred quickly enough to community or other services. The discharge summary should be shared with the patient and if appropriate, the carer. A key component of effective care is planning for a patient's discharge from hospital. There are a number of patients who are discharged from hospital who have care needs that are ongoing, and these must be met in the community. Care needs can include:

- The use of specialised equipment at home, for example, a hospital-type bed
- Daily support from carers to assist with completion of the activities of living
- Regular visits from district nurses to administer medication or to carry out wound care.

When there is a specific targeted discharge date and time, this has the potential to reduce a patient's length of stay, prevent emergency readmissions and reduce the pressure on hospital beds. This is the case for all patients, be it those who are having day surgery through to those with more complex needs.

Discharge planning

Discharge planning is seen as the process by which the hospital team considers the support that the patient might require in the community, referring patients to these services and liaising with these services to manage the patient's discharge.

Discharge should not be seen as an isolated event it is a coordinated, patient-focused and transparent process. Patients, family and carers are treated with dignity and respect, and they are encouraged to be actively engaged in all plans and decisions about their future care. In the community, a wide variety of care packages are available. However, planning must be done before the patient's return to ensure that there is no gap in the provision of care between the discharge from hospital and the commencement of community services.

To ensure a high-quality service, discharge planning should, wherever possible, begin prior to the patient being admitted for care. Discharge planning encompasses the physical, psychological and social aspects of the individual patient and their family. The safety and effectiveness of care is often dependent upon accurate and appropriate communication. This is an important issue in discharge planning that needs to be given much attention. There is very often a wide range of people involved in the discharge process (see Figure 67.1).

Transfer of care

When people move between various health and care settings, information about their care, their health and well-being and medications, for example, should be shared with all the professionals who have been and will continue to be involved in their care. This needs to be done in a manner which protects the privacy and confidentiality of patients.

Standardised information has to be gathered and shared in health and care records in order to ensure that the right data can flow digitally across health and social care, supporting the provision of high-quality, timely and efficient care. The inability to share information can lead to unnecessary duplication of tests and delays in patients receiving appropriate treatment. This can cause potentially serious consequences which compromise both the safety and quality of care provided. Information should accompany the patient along the entire care pathway. Contemporary clinical practice seeks to reduce a patient's time in an acute hospital to a minimum.

Hospital passport

A hospital passport (a summary care record) provides important information about a patient (they are often used with people having a learning disability). The information includes personal details, the type of medication being taken and any pre-existing health conditions. The passport also provides information about how a person communicates and what their likes and dislikes are. This can include communication aids, and how they can be used so that health staff can clearly communicate with the person. In addition, they can also indicate how the person expresses happiness, sadness, pain and discomfort. This allows Nursing Associates and other staff to understand the needs of the individual and to help them make the necessary reasonable adjustments that may be required to offer care and treatment.

Appendix (i) Annexes A and B (NMC, 2018)

Annexe A: Communication and relationship management skills

Introduction

In order to meet the proficiency outcomes outlined in the main body of this document, Nursing Associates must be able to demonstrate the communication and relationship management skills described in this annexe at the point of registration.

The ability to communicate effectively, with sensitivity and compassion, and to manage relationships with people is central to the provision of high quality person-centred care. These competencies must be demonstrated in practice settings and adapted to meet the needs of people across their lifespan. Nursing Associates need a diverse range of communication skills and strategies to ensure that individuals, their families and carers are supported to be actively involved in their own care wherever appropriate, and that they are kept informed and well prepared.

It will be important for Nursing Associates to demonstrate cultural awareness when caring for people and to ensure that the needs, priorities, expertise and preferences of people are always valued and taken into account.

Where people have special communication needs or a disability, it is essential that Nursing Associates make reasonable adjustments. This means they'll be able to provide and share information in a way that promotes good health and health outcomes and does not prevent people from having equal access to the highest quality of care.

The skills listed below are those that all Nursing Associates are expected to demonstrate at the point of registration.

At the point of registration, the Nursing Associate will be able to safely demonstrate the following skills:

1 Underpinning communication skills for providing and monitoring care:

1.1 actively listen, recognise and respond to verbal and non-verbal cues

1.2 use prompts and positive verbal and non-verbal reinforcement

1.3 use appropriate non-verbal communication including touch, eye contact and personal space

1.4 make appropriate use of open and closed questioning

1.5 speak clearly and accurately

1.6 use caring conversation techniques

1.7 check understanding and use clarification techniques

1.8 be aware of the possibility of own unconscious bias in communication encounters

1.9 write accurate, clear, legible records and documentation

1.10 clearly record digital information and data

1.11 provide clear verbal, digital or written information and instructions when sharing information, delegating or handing over responsibility for care

1.12 recognise the need for translator services and material

1.13 use age appropriate communication techniques.

2 Communication skills for supporting people to prevent ill health and manage their health challenges:

2.1 effectively share information and check understanding about:

- preventative health behaviours that help people to make lifestyle choices and improve their own health and wellbeing
- a range of common conditions including: anxiety, depression, memory loss, diabetes, dementia, respiratory disease, cardiac disease, neurological disease, cancer, skin problems, immune deficiencies, psychosis, stroke and arthritis in accordance with care plans

2.2 clearly and confidently explain to the individual and family how their lifestyle choices may influence their health. This includes the impact of common health risk behaviours including smoking, diet, sexual practice, alcohol and substance use

2.3 use appropriate materials, making reasonable adjustments where appropriate to support people's understanding of what may have caused their health condition and the implications of their care and treatment

2.4 use repetition and positive reinforcement strategies

2.5 recognise and accommodate sensory impairments during all communications

2.6 support and monitor the use of personal communication aids

2.7 address and respond to people's questions, recognising when to refer to others in order to provide accurate responses

2.8 identify the need for and manage a range of alternative communication techniques

2.9 engage in difficult conversations with support from others, helping people who are feeling emotionally or physically vulnerable or in distress, conveying compassion and sensitivity.

3 Communication skills and approaches for providing therapeutic interventions:

3.1 identify the need for and use appropriate approaches to develop therapeutic relationships with people

3.2 demonstrate the use of a variety of effective communication strategies:

- reassurance and affirmation
- de-escalation strategies and techniques
- distraction and diversion strategies
- positive behaviour support approaches.

4 Communication skills for working in professional teams:

Demonstrate effective skills when working in teams through:

4.1 active listening when receiving feedback and when dealing with team members' concerns and anxieties

4.2 timely and appropriate escalation

4.3 being a calm presence when exposed to situations involving conflict

The Nursing Associate at a Glance, First Edition. Ian Peate.
© 2021 John Wiley & Sons Ltd. Published 2021 by John Wiley & Sons Ltd.

4.4 being assertive when required

4.5 using de-escalation strategies and techniques when dealing with conflict.

5 Demonstrate effective supervision skills by providing:

5.1 clear instructions and explanations when supervising others

5.2 clear instructions and checking understanding when delegating care responsibilities to others

5.3 clear constructive feedback in relation to care delivered by others

5.4 encouragement to colleagues that helps them to reflect on their practice.

Annexe B: Procedures to be undertaken by the Nursing Associate

Introduction

In order to meet the proficiency outcomes outlined in the main body of this document, Nursing Associates must be able to carry out the procedures described in this annexe at the point of their registration. Nursing Associates are required to demonstrate an awareness of how requirements for procedures may vary across different health and care settings. As the Nursing Associate role is generic, students may demonstrate the ability to carry out procedures in any appropriate context, and there is no expectation that this must be demonstrated in every health and care setting. Ideally students will demonstrate skills in a practice setting, but where necessary some procedures may be demonstrated through simulation.

Nursing Associates are expected to apply evidence based best practice across all procedures. The ability to carry out these procedures, safely, effectively, with sensitivity and compassion (while demonstrating the communication and relationship management skills described in Annexe A) is crucial to the provision of person-centred care. These procedures must be demonstrated with an awareness of variations required for different practice settings and for people across their lifespan. They must be carried out in a way that reflects cultural awareness and ensures that the needs, priorities, expertise and preferences of people are always valued and taken into account.

At the point of registration, the Nursing Associate will be able to safely demonstrate the following procedures:

Part 1: Procedures to enable effective monitoring of a person's condition

1 Demonstrate effective approaches to monitoring signs and symptoms of physical, mental, cognitive, behavioural and emotional distress, deterioration and improvement:

1.1 accurately measure weight and height, calculate body mass index and recognise healthy ranges and clinically significant low/high readings

1.2 use manual techniques and devices to take, record and interpret vital signs including temperature, pulse, respiration (TPR), blood pressure (BP) and pulse oximetry in order to identify signs of improvement, deterioration or concern

1.3 undertake venepuncture and routine ECG recording

1.4 measure and interpret blood glucose levels

1.5 collect and observe sputum, urine, stool and vomit specimens, interpreting findings and reporting as appropriate

1.6 recognise and escalate signs of all forms of abuse

1.7 recognise and escalate signs of self-harm and/or suicidal ideation

1.8 undertake and interpret neurological observations

1.9 recognise signs of mental and emotional distress including agitation, or vulnerability

1.10 administer basic mental health first aid

1.11 recognise emergency situations and administer basic physical first aid, including basic life support.

Part 2: Procedures for provision of person-centred nursing care

2 Provide support in meeting the needs of people in relation to rest, sleep, comfort and the maintenance of dignity:

2.1 observe and monitor comfort and pain levels and rest and sleep patterns

2.2 use appropriate bed-making techniques, including those required for people who are unconscious or who have limited mobility

2.3 use appropriate positioning and pressure relieving techniques

2.4 take appropriate action to ensure privacy and dignity at all times

2.5 appropriate action to reduce or minimise pain or discomfort

2.6 support people to reduce fatigue, minimise insomnia and take appropriate rest.

3 Provide care and support with hygiene and the maintenance of skin integrity:

3.1 observe and reassess skin and hygiene status using contemporary approaches to determine the need for support and ongoing intervention.

3.2 identify the need for and provide appropriate assistance with washing, bathing, shaving and dressing

3.3 identify the need for and provide appropriate oral, dental, eye and nail care and suggest to others when an onward referral is needed

3.4 prevent and manage skin breakdown through appropriate use of products

3.5 Identify and manage skin irritations and rashes

3.6 monitor wounds and undertake wound care using appropriate evidence-based techniques.

4 Provide support with nutrition and hydration:

4.1 use contemporary nutritional assessment tools

4.2 assist with feeding and drinking and use appropriate feeding and drinking aids

4.3 record fluid intake and output to identify signs of dehydration or fluid retention and escalate as necessary

4.4 support the delivery of artificial nutrition and hydration using oral and enteral routes.

5 Provide support with maintaining bladder and bowel health:

5.1 observe and monitor the level of urinary and bowel continence to determine the need for ongoing support and intervention, the level of independence and self-management of care that an individual can manage

5.2 assist with toileting, maintaining dignity and privacy and use appropriate continence products

5.3 care for and manage catheters for all genders

5.4 recognise bladder and bowel patterns to identify and respond to incontinence, constipation, diarrhoea and urinary and faecal retention.

6 Provide support with mobility and safety:

6.1 use appropriate risk assessment tools to determine the ongoing need for support and intervention, the level of independence and self-care that an individual can manage

6.2 use appropriate assessment tools to determine, manage and escalate the ongoing risk of falls

6.3 use a range of contemporary moving and handling techniques and mobility aids

6.4 use appropriate moving and handling equipment to support people with impaired mobility.

7 Provide support with respiratory care:

7.1 manage the administration of oxygen using a range of routes and approaches

7.2 take and be able to identify normal peak flow and oximetry measurements

7.3 use appropriate nasal and oral suctioning techniques

7.4 manage inhalation, humidifier and nebuliser devices.

8 Preventing and managing infection:

8.1 observe and respond rapidly to potential infection risks using best practice guidelines

8.2 use standard precautions protocols

8.3 use aseptic, non-touch techniques

8.4 use appropriate personal protection equipment

8.5 implement isolation procedures

8.6 use hand hygiene techniques

8.7 safely decontaminate equipment and environment

8.8 safely handle waste, laundry and sharps.

9 Meeting needs for care and support at the end of life:

9.1 recognise and take immediate steps to respond appropriately to uncontrolled symptoms and signs of distress including pain, nausea, thirst, constipation, restlessness, agitation, anxiety and depression

9.2 review preferences and care priorities of the dying person and their family and carers, and ensure changes are communicated as appropriate

9.3 provide care for the deceased person and the bereaved respecting cultural requirements and protocols.

10 Procedural competencies required for administering medicines safely:

10.1 continually assess people receiving care and their ongoing ability to self-administer their own medications. Know when and how to escalate any concerns

10.2 undertake accurate drug calculations for a range of medications

10.3 exercise professional accountability in ensuring the safe administration of medicines to those receiving care

10.4 administer medication via oral, topical and inhalation routes

10.5 administer injections using subcutaneous and intramuscular routes and manage injection equipment

10.6 administer and monitor medications using enteral equipment

10.7 administer enemas and suppositories

10.8 manage and monitor effectiveness of symptom relief medication

10.9 recognise and respond to adverse or abnormal reactions to medications, and when and how to escalate any concerns

10.10 undertake safe storage, transportation and disposal of medicinal products.

References and bibliography

Chapter 1

Nursing and Midwifery Council (2018). The Code. Professional standards of practice and behaviour for nurses, midwives and nursing associates. https://www.nmc.org.uk/globalassets/sitedocuments/nmc-publications/nmc-code.pdf. Last accessed December 2019.

Nursing and Midwifery Council (2018). Standards of proficiency for nursing associates. https://www.nmc.org.uk/globalassets/sitedocuments/education-standards/nursing-associates-proficiency-standards.pdf. Last accessed December 2019.

Chapter 2

Avery, G. (2017). *Law and Ethics in Nursing and Health Care: An Introduction*, 2nd Ed. Sage: London.

Gates, B., Fearns, D. and Welch, J. (2015). *Learning Disabilities Nursing at a Glance*. Wiley. Oxford

Chapter 3

Nursing and Midwifery Council and General Medical Council (2015). Openness and honesty when things go wrong. The professional duty of candour. https://www.nmc.org.uk/globalassets/sitedocuments/nmc-publications/openness-and-honesty-professional-duty-of-candour.pdf. Last accessed December 2019.

Professional Standards Authority (2019). Telling patients the truth when something goes wrong. https://www.professionalstandards.org.uk/docs/default-source/publications/research-paper/telling-patients-the-truth-when-something-goes-wrong---how-have-professional-regulators-encouraged-professionals-to-be-candid-to-patients.pdf?sfvrsn=100f7520_6. Last accessed December 2019.

Wijesuriya, J.D. and Walker, D. (2017). Duty of candour: A statutory obligation or just the right thing to do?" *British Journal of Anaesthesia* 119(2): 175–178.

Chapter 4

Asamoah-Danso, T. and Mistry, A. (2020). #BlackLivesMatter 2020. *Journal of Paramedic Practice* 12(7): 290.

Royal College of Nursing (2020). Discrimination. https://www.rcn.org.uk/get-help/rcn-advice/discrimination. Last accessed July 2020.

University of Bristol (2019). Learning disability mortality review (LeDeR Programme). https://www.hqip.org.uk/wp-content/uploads/2019/05/LeDeR-Annual-Report-Final-21-May-2019.pdf. Last accessed July 2020.

Chapter 5

Royal College of Nursing (2015). Health workplace toolkit. https://www.rcn.org.uk/professional-development/publications/pub-004964. Last accessed December 2019.

UNISON (2019). Stress. https://www.unison.org.uk/get-help/knowledge/health-and-safety/stress/.

Chapter 6

Nursing and Midwifery Council (2019). Guidance on health and character. https://www.nmc.org.uk/globalassets/sitedocuments/registration/guidance-on-health-and-character.pdf. Last accessed December 2019.

University College London (2014). Local action on health inequalities: building children and young people's resilience in schools. http://www.instituteofhealthequity.org/resources-reports/building-children-and-young-peoples-resilience-in-schools/evidence-review-2-building-childrens-and-young-peoples-resilience-in-schools.pdf. Last accessed December 2019.

World Health Organization (2019). Constitution. https://www.who.int/about/who-we-are/constitution. Last accessed December 2019.

Chapter 7

Glasper, A. and Rees, C. (eds) (2017). *Nursing and Healthcare Research At A Glance*. Wiley: Oxford.

Grove, S. (2019). *Understanding Nursing Research: Building an Evidence Based Practice*, 7th Ed. Elsevier: Edinburgh.

Heaslip, V. (2019). *Research and Evidence Base Practice: for Nursing, Health and Social Care Students*. Lantern: Banbury.

Chapter 8

Codier, E. and Codier, D. (2017). Could emotional intelligence make patients safer? *American Journal of Nursing* 7(117): 58–62.

Heffernan, M., Griffin, M., McNulty, R. and Fitzpatrick, J. (2010). Self compassion and emotional intelligence in nurses. *International Journal of Nursing Practice* 16: 366–373.

Salovery, P. and Mayer, J. (1990). Emotional intelligence. *Imagination Cognition and Personality* 9: 85–211.

Chapter 9

Nursing and Midwifery Council (2018). The Code. Professional standards of practice and behaviour for nurses, midwives and nursing associates. https://www.nmc.org.uk/globalassets/sitedocuments/nmc-publications/nmc-code.pdf. Last accessed January 2020.

Royal College of Nursing (2016). Why communication important. https://rcni.com/hosted-content/rcn/first-steps/why-communication-important. Last accessed January 2020.

Webb, L. (2011). *Nursing: Communication Skills in Practice*. Oxford University Press: Oxford.

Chapter 10

Nursing and Midwifery Board of Ireland (2013). Guidance to nurses and midwives on social media and social networking. https://www.ul.ie/nm/sites/default/files/Guidance%20to%20Nurses%20%26%20Midwives%20on%20Social%20Media%20%2B%20Social%20Networking.pdf. Last accessed January 2020.

Nursing and Midwifery Council (2019). Guidance on using social media responsibility. https://www.nmc.org.uk/globalassets/sitedocuments/nmc-publications/social-media-guidance.pdf. Last accessed January 2020.

Chapter 11

Health Education England (2018). Diversity and inclusion. Our strategic framework 2018–2022. https://www.hee.nhs.uk/sites/default/files/documents/Diversity%20and%20Inclusion%20-%20Our%20Strategic%20Framework.pdf. Last accessed January 2020.

Health Foundation (2016). Person-centred care made simple. What everyone should know about person-centred care. https://www.health.org.uk/sites/default/files/PersonCentredCareMadeSimple_0.pdf. Last accessed February 2020.

Picker Institute Europe (2019). Influence, inspire, empower. Impact report 2018-2019. https://www.picker.org/wp-content/uploads/2020/01/Picker-Impact-Report_2018-2019_Web_spreads-3.pdf. Last accessed February 2020.

Scottish Human Rights Commission (2020). PANEL principles. http://www.scottishhumanrights.com/rights-in-practice/human-rights-based-approach/#the-panel-principles-1210. Last accessed February 2020.

Chapter 12

Social Care Wales (2017). Openness and honesty when things go wrong: The professional duty of candour. Explanatory guidance for social care professionals registered with social care Wales. https://socialcare.wales/cms:assets/file-uploads/SCW-DutyofCandour-ENG-V01.pdf. Last accessed March 2020.

Nursing and Midwifery Council and General Medical Council (2015). Openness and honesty when things go wrong: The professional duty of candour. https://www.gmc-uk.org/-/media/documents/openness-and-honesty-when-things-go-wrong--the-professional-duty-of-cand____pdf-61540594.pdf. Last accessed March 2020.

Royal College of Nursing (2020). Patient safety and human factors. https://www.rcn.org.uk/clinical-topics/patient-safety-and-human-factors. Last accessed March 2020.

Chapter 13

Royal College of Nursing (2018. Every nurse an e-nurse. https://www.rcn.org.uk/professional-development/publications/pdf-007013. Last accessed March 2020.

Royal College of Nursing (2019). Digital skills. https://www.rcn.org.uk/clinical-topics/ehealth/digital-skills. Last accessed March 2020.

Royal College of Nursing (2020). Safety in numbers. https://www.rcn.org.uk/clinical-topics/safety-in-numbers. Last accessed March 2020.

Chapter 14

Griffith, R.A. and Dowie, I. (2019). *Dimond's Legal Aspects of Nursing: A Definitive Guide to Law for Nurses*, 8th Ed. Pearson: Harlow.

Merrix, P. and Lillyman, S. (2014) *Nursing and Health Survival Guide: Record Keeping*. Routledge: London.

Peate, I. and Stevens, M. (2020). *Wound Care at a Glance*, 2nd Ed. Wiley: Oxford.

Chapter 15

Bulman, C., Lathlean, J. and Gobbi, M. (2012). The concept of reflection in nursing: Qualitative findings on student and teacher perspectives. *Nurse Education Today* 32(5): e8–13 https://www.sciencedirect.com/science/article/abs/pii/S0260691711002693?via%3Dihub.

Rolfe, G., Jasper, M., and Freshwater, D. (2010). *Critical Reflection in Practice*, 2nd Ed. Palgrave: Macmillan Basingstoke.

Schön, D.A. (1983). *The Reflective Practitioner: How Professionals Think in Action*. Temple Smith: London.

Chapter 16

International Council of Nurses (2020). 2020 International Year of the Nurse and Midwife. https://www.icn.ch/news/2020-international-year-nurse-and-midwife-catalyst-brighter-future-health-around-globe. Last accessed March 2020.

Nursing and Midwifery Council (2018). The code. Professional standards of practice and behaviour for nurses, midwives and nursing associates. https://www.nmc.org.uk/globalassets/sitedocuments/nmc-publications/nmc-code.pdf. Last accessed March 2020.

Royal College of Nursing (2013). Engaging with the principles of nursing practice. Guide reflection for nursing students. https://www.rcn.org.uk/professional-development/publications/pub-004432. Last accessed March 2020.

Chapter 17

Hubley, J. (2013). *Practical Health Promotion*, 2nd Ed. Polity Press: Cambridge.

Prochaska, J.O. and DiCliemente, C.C. (1986). "Towards a Comprehensive Model of Change" Ch 1 in Treating Addictive Behaviors: Processes of Change (eds. Miller, W. R. and Heather, N.), 3–27. Plenum, New York.

Wild, K, (2018). Health Promotion. Ch 3 in *Nursing Practice. Knowledge and Care*, 2nd Ed. (eds. Peate, I. and Wild, K.), 50–70. Wiley: Oxford.

Chapter 18

Gochman, D.S. (ed.) (1997). *Handbook of Health Behavior Research* (vols 1–4). Plenum: New York.

National Institute for Health and Care Excellence (2014). Behaviour change. Individual approaches. Nice Guidelines (PH49). https://www.nice.org.uk/guidance/ph49. Last accessed March 2020.

Behavioural Insights Team (2020). http://www.behaviouralinsights.co.uk/. Last accessed March 2020.

Chapter 19

NHS England (2017). 100,000 Genomes Project paving the way to Personalised Medicine. https://webarchive.nationalarchives.gov.uk/20171102123005/https://www.england.nhs.uk/publication/100000-genomes-project-paving-the-way-to-personalised-medicine/. Last accessed March 2020.

Somerville, M., Kumaran, K. and Anderson, R. (2012). *Public Health and Epidemiology at a Glance*, 2nd Ed. Wiley: Oxford.

Chapter 20

King's Fund (2020). What are health inequalities. https://www.kingsfund.org.uk/publications/what-are-health-inequalities. Last accessed Match 2020.

Public Health England (2018). *Local Action on Health Inequalities Understanding and Reducing Ethnic Inequalities in Health*. PHE: London.

NHS England and Public Health England (ND). Reducing health inequalities resources. https://www.england.nhs.uk/about/equality/equality-hub/resources/. Last accessed March 2020.

Chapter 21

Bellis, M.A., Ashton, K., Hughes, K. et al (2016). Adverse childhood experiences (ACEs) in Wales and their impact on health in the adult population: Mariana Dyakova. *European Journal of Public Health* 26(Suppl. 1), ckw167.009. https://doi.org/10.1093/eurpub/ckw167.009

Felitti, V.J., Ana, R.F., Nordenberg, D. et al. (1998). Relationship of childhood abuse and household dysfunction to many of the leading causes of death in adults. The Adverse Childhood Experiences (ACE) study. *American Journal of Preventative Medicine* 14(4): 245–258.

Harvard University Centre for the Developing Child (2020). Toxic stress. https://developingchild.harvard.edu/science/key-concepts/toxic-stress/. Last accessed March 2020.

Public Health Wales NHS Trust (2015). Adverse childhood experiences and their impact on health-harming behaviours in the Welsh adult population. http://www2.nphs.wales.nhs.uk:8080/PRIDDocs.nsf/7c21215d6d0c613e80256f490030c05a/d488a3852491bc1d80257f370038919e/$FILE/ACE%20Report%20FINAL%20(E).pdf. Last accessed March 2020.

Chapter 22

Nutbeam, D. (2000). Health literacy as a public health goal: A challenge for contemporary health education and communication strategies into the 21st century. Health Promotion International 15(3): 259–267.

Public Health England (2015). Local action on health inequalities. Improving health literacy to reduce health inequalities. https://assets.publishing.service.gov.uk/government/uploads/system/uploads/attachment_data/file/460710/4b_Health_Literacy-Briefing.pdf. Last accessed April 2020.

World Health Organization (2015). Health literacy toolkit for low- and middle-Income countries. https://apps.who.int/iris/bitstream/handle/10665/205244/B5148.pdf?sequence=1&isAllowed=y. Last accessed March 2020.

Chapter 23

Peate, I. (2019). NHS screening programmes. *British Journal of Healthcare Assistants* 13(8): 378–381.

Public Health England (2017). NHS Screening Programme Available in England. https://assets.publishing.service.gov.uk/government/uploads/system/uploads/attachment_data/file/661677/NHS_Screening_Programmes_in_England_2016_to_2017_web_version_final.pdf. Last accessed April 2020.

Sense About Science (2015). Making Sense of Screening. Weighing up the Benefits and Harms of Health Screening Programmes, 2nd Ed. https://senseaboutscience.org/activities/making-sense-of-screening/. April 2020.

Chapter 24

National Health Service (2019). NHS vaccinations and when to have them. https://www.nhs.uk/conditions/vaccinations/nhs-vaccinations-and-when-to-have-them/. Last accessed April 2020.

Oxford Vaccine Group (2019). Vaccine Knowledge Project. https://vk.ovg.ox.ac.uk/vk/uk-schedule. Last accessed April 2020.

UK Government (Various). *Immunisation Against Infectious Disease (Green Book).* https://www.gov.uk/government/collections/immunisation-against-infectious-disease-the-green-book#the-green-book. Last accessed April 2020.

Chapter 25

Health care without avoidable infections. The critical role of infection prevention and control. https://apps.who.int/iris/bitstream/handle/10665/246235/WHO-HIS-SDS-2016.10-eng.pdf;jsessionid=84350E6CE688A22044B0E607D9EF1D59?sequence=1. Last accessed April 2020.

Royal College of Nursing (2017). Essential practice for infection prevention and control. guidance for nursing staff. https://www.rcn.org.uk/professional-development/publications/pub-005940. Last accessed April 2020.

Weston, D., Burgess, A. and Roberts, S. (2017). *Infection Prevention and Control at a Glance.* Wiley: Oxford.

Chapter 26

Erikson, E.H. (1963). *Childhood and Society.* Norton and Company: New York.

Public Health England (2019). Health matters: Prevention - A life course approach. https://publichealthmatters.blog.gov.uk/2019/05/23/health-matters-prevention-a-life-course-approach/. Last accessed April 2020.

World Health Organization (2017). A life-course approach to health: Synergy with sustainable development goals. https://www.who.int/bulletin/volumes/96/1/17-198358/en/. Last accessed April 2020.

Chapter 27

Peate, I. (ed.) (2020). *Fundamentals of Pathophysiology for Nursing and Healthcare Students*, 4th Ed. Wiley: Oxford.

Peate, I. and Evans, S. (eds) (2020). *Fundamentals of Anatomy and Physiology for Nursing and Healthcare Students*, 3rd Ed. Wiley: Oxford.

Chapter 28

HM Government and Department of Health (2011). No health without mental health. https://assets.publishing.service.gov.uk/government/uploads/system/uploads/attachment_data/file/138253/dh_124058.pdf. Last accessed April 2020.

Nursing, Midwifery and Allied Health Professions Policy Unit (2016). Improving the physical health of people with mental health problems: actions for mental health nurses. https://assets.publishing.service.gov.uk/government/uploads/system/uploads/attachment_data/file/532253/JRA_Physical_Health_revised.pdf. Last accessed April 2020.

Royal College of Nursing (2019). *Parity of Esteem – Delivering Physical Health Equality for Those with Serious Mental Health Needs.* RCN: London.

Chapter 29

Coulter, A. (2018). How to provide patients with the right information to make informed decisions. *The Pharmaceutical Journal*, June. https://www.pharmaceutical-journal.com/acute-pain/how-to-provide-patients-with-the-right-information-to-make-informed-decisions/20204936.article?firstPass=false. Last accessed May 2020.

NHS Improvement (ND). Patient information. https://improvement.nhs.uk/documents/2139/patient-information.pdf. Last accessed May 2020.

NHS Digital (2020). A to Z of NHS health writing. https://service-manual.nhs.uk/content/a-to-z-of-nhs-health-writing. Last accessed May 2020.

Chapter 30

Coulter, A. and Collins, A. (2011). Making shared decision making a reality. No decision about me without me. https://www.kingsfund.org.uk/sites/default/files/Making-shared-decision-making-a-reality-paper-Angela-Coulter-Alf-Collins-July-2011_0.pdf. Last accessed May 2020.

National Institute for Health and Care Excellence (2020). Shared decision making. https://www.nice.org.uk/about/what-we-do/our-programmes/nice-guidance/nice-guidelines/shared-decision-making. Last accessed May 2020.

NHS England and NHS Improvement (2019). Shared decision. Making summary guide. https://www.england.nhs.uk/wp-content/uploads/2019/01/shared-decision-making-summary-guide-v1.pdf. Last accessed May 2020.

Chapter 31

Felton, M. (2017). Recognising signs and symptoms of patient deterioration. *Emergency Nurse* 20(8): 23–27.

National Institute for Health and Clinical Excellence (2007). Acutely Ill adults in hospital: Recognising and responding to deterioration. https://www.nice.org.uk/guidance/cg50/resources/acutely-ill-adults-in-hospital-recognising-and-responding-to-deterioration-pdf-975500772037. Last accessed May 2020.

Scottish Intercollegiate Guidelines Network (2014). Care of deteriorating patients. Consensus recommendations. https://www.sign.ac.uk/assets/sign139.pdf. Last accessed May 2020.

Chapter 32

National Dignity Campaign (2016). Dignity in care campaign leaflet and role descriptors. https://www.dignityincare.org.uk/Resources/Type/Dignity-in-Care-Campaign-leaflet-and-role-descriptors/. Last accessed May 2020.

NHS (2015). NHS constitution the NHS belongs to us all. https://assets.publishing.service.gov.uk/government/uploads/system/uploads/attachment_data/file/480482/NHS_Constitution_WEB.pdf. Last accessed May 2020.

NHS England and NHS Improvement (2019). The NHS Patient Safety Strategy. Safer culture, safer systems, safer patients. https://improvement.nhs.uk/documents/5472/190708_Patient_Safety_Strategy_for_website_v4.pdf. Last accessed May 2020.

National Sleep Foundation (2020). How much sleep do we really need? https://www.sleepfoundation.org/articles/how-much-sleep-do-we-really-need. Last accessed May 2020.

Chapter 33

Anderson, L. (2017). Assisting patients with eating and drinking to prevent malnutrition. *Nursing Times* 113(11): 23–25. https://www.nursingtimes.net/clinical-archive/nutrition/assisting-patients-with-eating-and-drinking-to-prevent-malnutrition-09-10-2017/. Last accessed May 2020.

Cunningham, S. (2020). *Nursing Skills in Nutrition, Hydration and Elimination.* Routledge: London.

National Institute for Health and Care Excellence (2017). Nutrition support in adults. https://www.nice.org.uk/guidance/qs24/resources/nutrition-support-in-adults-pdf-2098545777349. Last accessed May 2020.

Chapter 34

Giddens, J.F. (2017). *Concepts for Nursing Practice*, 2nd Ed. Elsevier: St Louis.

Peate, I. and Wild, K. (eds) (2018). *Nursing Practice Knowledge and Care*, 2nd Ed. Wiley: Oxford.

Peate, I. (ed.) (2020). *Alexander's Nursing Practice: Hospital and Home*, 5th Ed. Elsevier: London.

Chapter 35

Gluyas, H. (2017). Errors in the nursing management of a deteriorating patient. *Nursing Standard* 32(12): 41–50. doi: 10.7748/ns.2017.e10874

Vincent, J.L., Einav, S., Pearse, R. et al (2018). Improving detection of patient deterioration in the general hospital ward environment. *European Journal of Anaesthesiology* 55(5): 325–333. doi: 10.1097/ EJA.0000000000000798

National Institute for Health and Clinical Excellence (2007). Acutely Ill adults in hospital: Recognising and responding to deterioration. https://www.nice.org.uk/guidance/cg50/resources/acutely-ill-adults-in-hospital-recognising-and-responding-to-deterioration-pdf-975500772037. Last accessed May 2020.

Chapter 36

National Institute for Health and Clinical Excellence (2019a). Generalised anxiety disorder and panic disorder in adults: management. https://www.nice.org.uk/guidance/cg113/chapter/introduction. Last accessed May 2020.

National Institute for Health and Clinical Excellence (2019b). Delirium: Prevention, diagnosis and management. https://www.nice.org.uk/guidance/CG103/chapter/introduction. Last accessed May 2020.

NHS Improvement (ND). Confusion care pathway. https://improvement.nhs.uk/resources/confusion-care-pathway/. Last accessed May 2020.

Chapter 37

British Pain Society (2015). Understanding and managing long-term pain. Information for people in pain. https://www.britishpainsociety.org/static/uploads/resources/files/Understanding_and_Managing_Long-term_Pain_Final2015.pdf Last accessed May 2020.

Cox, F. (2018). Advances in the pharmacological management of acute and chronic pain. Nursing Standar*d* 33(3): 37–42. doi: 10.7748/ ns.2018.e11191.

McGann, K. (2007). *Fundamental Aspects of Pain Assessment and Management*. Quay Books: Gateshead.

Chapter 38

Department of Health. (2012). End of life care strategy. Fourth annual report. https://www.gov.uk/government/publications/end-of-life-care-strategy-fourth-annual-report. Last accessed May 2020.

NHS Improving Quality *(*2014*)*. End of life care. Achieving quality in hostels and for homeless people – a route to success. https://www.england.nhs.uk/improvement-hub/wp-content/uploads/sites/44/2017/11/End-of-Life-Care-Hostels-and-Homeless-People.pdf. Last accessed May 2020.

National Institute for Health and Care Excellence (2015). Care of dying adults in the last days of life. https://www.nice.org.uk/guidance/ng31/resources/care-of-dying-adults-in-the-last-days-of-life-pdf-1837387324357. Last accessed May 2020.

Chapter 39

Skills for Health (2017). End of life care. Core skills education and training framework. https://www.skillsforhealth.org.uk/images/services/cstf/EoLC%20-%20Core%20Skills%20Training%20Framework.pdf?s=form. Last accessed May 2020.

National Institute for Health and Care Excellence (2015). End of life care for adults in the last days of life. https://www.nice.org.uk/guidance/qs13/resources/end-of-life-care-for-adults-pdf-2098483631557. Last accessed May 2020.

Royal College of Nursing (2020). End of life care. https://www.rcn.org.uk/clinical-topics/end-of-life-care. Last accessed May 2020.

Chapter 40

National Institute for Health and Care Excellence (2015). Medicines optimisation: The safe and effective use of medicines to enable the best possible outcomes. https://www.nice.org.uk/guidance/ng5/resources/medicines-optimisation-the-safe-and-effective-use-of-medicines-to-enable-the-best-possible-outcomes-pdf-51041805253. Last accessed May 2020.

Royal College of Nursing (2020). *Medicines Management: An Overview for Nursing*. Royal College of Nursing: London.

Royal Pharmaceutical Society (2013). Medicines optimisation: Helping patient to make the most of medicines. https://www.rpharms.com/Portals/0/RPS%20document%20library/Open%20access/Policy/helping-patients-make-the-most-of-their-medicines.pdf. Last accessed May 2020.

Chapter 41

Deslandes, P. (2020). *Rapid Medicines Management for Healthcare Professionals*. Wiley: Oxford.

Joint Formulary Committee (2019). *British National Formulary: How to use BNF Publications Online*. London: Joint Formulary Committee. https://bnf.nice.org.uk/about/how-to-use-bnf-publications-online.html. Last accessed May 2020.

World Health Organization (2019). Pharmacovigilance. https://www.who.int/medicines/areas/quality_safety/safety_efficacy/pharmvigi/en/. Last accessed May 2020.

Chapter 42

Lawson, E. and Hennefer, D.L. (2010). *Medicines Management in Adult Nursing*. Exeter: Learning Matters.

Peate, I. and Hill, B. (2020). *Fundamentals of Pharmacology for Nursing and Health Care Students*. Wiley: Oxford.

Young, S. (2016). *Medicines Management for Nurses at a Glance*. Wiley: Oxford.

Chapter 43

Care Quality Commission (2016). Better care in my hands: A review of how people are involved in their care. https://www.cqc.org.uk/sites/default/files/20160519_Better_care_in_my_hands_FINAL.pdf. Last accessed May 2020.

Department of Health (2015). The NHS constitution: The NHS belongs to us. https://assets.publishing.service.gov.uk/government/uploads/system/uploads/attachment_data/file/480482/NHS_Constitution_WEB.pdf. Last accessed May 2020.

The Health Foundation (2016). Person- centred care made simple: What everyone should know about person-centred care. www.health.org.uk/sites/health/files/PersonCentredCareMadeSimple.pdf. Last accessed May 2020.

Chapter 44

British Geriatric Society (2018). Morbidity – Comorbidity and multimorbidity. What do they mean? https://www.bgs.org.uk/resources/morbidity-comorbidity-and-multimorbidity-what-do-they-mean. Last accessed June 2020.

National Institute for Health and Care Excellence (2016). Multimorbidity: Clinical assessment and management. https://www.nice.org.uk/guidance/ng56/resources/multimorbidity-clinical-assessment-and-management-pdf-1837516654789. Last accessed June 2020.

Chapter 45

Dimond, B. (2016). *Legal Aspects of Mental Capacity: A Practical Guide for Health and Social Care Professionals*, 2nd Ed. Wiley: Oxford.

Royal College of Nursing (2017). *Principles of Consent. Guidance for Nursing Staff*. RCN: London.

Social Care Institute for Excellence (2016). Mental Capacity Act 2005 at a glance. https://www.scie.org.uk/mca/introduction/mental-capacity-act-2005-at-a-glance. Last accessed June 2020.

Chapter 46

British Psychological Society (2017). Position statement: Understanding and preventing suicide: A psychological perspective. https://www.bps.org.uk/sites/www.bps.org.uk/files/Policy/Policy%20-%20Files/Understanding%20and%20preventing%20suicide%20-%20a%20psychological%20perspective.pdf. Last accessed June 2020.

HM Government (2017). *Preventing Suicide in England: Third Progress Report of the Cross-Government Outcomes Strategy to Save Lives*. Department of Health: London.

Mental Health Foundation (2006). *Truth Hurts. Report of the National Inquiry into Self-harm among Young People. Fact or Fiction?* Mental Health Foundation: London.

World Health Organization (2014). Preventing suicide: A global imperative. https://www.who.int/mental_health/suicideprevention/exe_summary_english.pdf?ua=1. Last accessed June 2020.

Chapter 47

Department of Health (2013). Information to share or not to share: Government response to the Caldicott review. https://assets.publishing.service.gov.uk/government/uploads/system/uploads/attachment_data/file/251750/9731-2901141-TSO-Caldicott-Government_Response_ACCESSIBLE.PDF. Last accessed June 2020.

HM Government (2018). Information sharing: advice for practitioners providing safeguarding services to children, young people, parents and carers. https://assets.publishing.service.gov.uk/government/uploads/system/uploads/attachment_data/file/721581/Information_sharing_advice_practitioners_safeguarding_services.pdf. Last accessed June 2020.

Royal College of Nursing (2019). *Principles of Consent: Guidance for Nursing Staff*. RCN: London.

Chapter 48

Nursing and Midwifery Council (2018). Standards of proficiency for nursing associates. https://www.nmc.org.uk/globalassets/sitedocuments/education-standards/nursing-associates-proficiency-standards.pdf. Last accessed June 2020.

Nursing and Midwifery Council (2019a). Blog: Role differences between nursing associates and nurses. https://www.nmc.org.uk/news/news-and-updates/blog-whats-a-nursing-associate/. Last accessed June 2020.

Nursing and Midwifery Council (2019b). Revalidation. https://www.nmc.org.uk/globalassets/sitedocuments/revalidation/how-to-revalidate-booklet.pdf. Last accessed June 2020.

Chapter 49

Maben, J., Peccei, R., Adams, M. et al. (2012). Patients' experiences of care and the influence of staff motivation, affect and wellbeing. Final Report. NIHR Service Delivery and Organisation Programme; 2012. http://www.netscc.ac.uk/hsdr/files/project/SDO_ES_08-1819-213_V01.pdf. Last accessed June 2020.

Royal College of Nursing (2015). Working with care – Improving working relationships in health and social care: Self-assessment tools for health and social care teams. https://www.rcn.org.uk/professional-development/publications/pub-004972. Last accessed June 2020.

Royal College of Nursing (2020). Accountability and delegation: A guide for the nursing team. https://www.rcn.org.uk/professional-development/accountability-and-delegation. Last accessed January 2020.

Chapter 50

Clinical Human Factors Group (2012). Never? https://drive.google.com/file/d/0B4dbLgB56hptOXNTUFlIVWJoWXM/view. Last accessed June 2020.

NHS Improvement (2018). Never events policy and framework. https://improvement.nhs.uk/documents/2265/Revised_Never_Events_policy_and_framework_FINAL.pdf.

Norris, B., Currie, L. and Lecko, C. (2012). The importance of applying human factors to nursing practice. *Nursing Standard* 26(32): 36–40. doi: 10.7748/ns2012.04.26.32.36.c9044

Chapter 51

Gretton, C. and Honeyman, M. (2016). The digital revolution: Eight technologies that will change health and care. https://www.kingsfund.org.uk/publications/eight-technologies-will-change-health-and-care. Last accessed June 2020.

Leary, A. (2018). Turning data into useful knowledge to improve patient care. *Nursing Management*. https://rcni.com/nursing-management/features/turning-data-useful-knowledge-to-improve-patient-care-132396#. Last accessed June 2020.

NHS England (2019). The Topol review. Preparing the healthcare workforce to deliver the digital future. An independent report on behalf of the secretary of state for health and social care. https://topol.hee.nhs.uk. Last accessed June 2020.

Chapter 52

Bramley, D. and Moody, D. (2016). Multimorbidity – the biggest clinical challenge facing the NHS? https://www.england.nhs.uk/blog/dawn-moody-david-bramley/. Last accessed July 2020.

Department of Health (ND). Comorbidities: A framework of principles for system-wide action https://assets.publishing.service.gov.uk/government/uploads/system/uploads/attachment_data/file/307143/Comorbidities_framework.pdf. Last accessed June 2020.

National Institute for Health and Care Excellence (2016). Multimorbidity: Clinical assessment and management. https://www.nice.org.uk/guidance/ng56/resources/multimorbidity-clinical-assessment-and-management-pdf-1837516654789. Last accessed June 2020.

Chapter 53

Mind Tools (2017). The Situation – Behavior – Impact™ feedback tool. https://www.mindtools.com/pages/article/situation-behavior-impact-feedback.htm. Last accessed July 2020.

Pendleton, D., Scofield, T., Tate, P. and Havelock P. (1984). *The Consultation: An Approach to Learning and Teaching*. Oxford University Press: Oxford.

Royal College of Nursing (2016). Patient/family complaints. https://rcni.com/hosted-content/rcn/first-steps/patient-family-complaints. Last accessed July 2020.

Chapter 54

NHS Employers (ND). How to ensure a quality training experience for trainee nursing associates? https://www.nhsemployers.org/nursingassociates/establishing-your-nursing-associate-training-programme/ensuring-a-quality-training-experience-for-trainee-nursing-associates. Last accessed July 2020.

Jack, K., Hampshire, C. and Chambers, A.J. (2017). The influence of role models in undergraduate nurse education. *Journal of Clinical Nursing* 26(23-24): 4707–4715.

Nursing and Midwifery Council (2019). Standards for student supervision and assessment. https://www.nmc.org.uk/standards-for-education-and-training/standards-for-student-supervision-and-assessment/. Last accessed July 2020.

Chapter 55

Stranks, J.W. (2016). *Health and Safety at Work: An Essential Guide for Managers*, 10th Ed. Kogan Page: London.

UNISON (2018). Violence at work it is not part of the job. https://www.unison.org.uk/get-help/knowledge/health-and-safety/. Last accessed July 2020.

Woodward, S. (2020). *Implementing Safety: Addressing Culture, Conditions and Values to Help People Work Safely*. Routledge: Abingdon.

Chapter 56

Benjamin, A. (2008). Audit: How to do it in practice. 336(7655): 1241–1245. doi: 10.1136/bmj.39527.628322.AD.

Healthcare Quality Improvement Partnership (2020a). "Documenting Local Clinical Audit: A Guide to Reporting and Recording" https://www.hqip.org.uk/wp-content/uploads/

2020/05/Final-Clinical-Audit-Reporting-guide-2020.pdf.
Last accessed July 2020.

Healthcare Quality Improvement Partnership (2020b). Best practice in clinical audit. https://www.hqip.org.uk/wp-content/uploads/2020/05/FINAL-Best-Practice-in-Clinical-Audit-2020.pdf. Last accessed July 2020.

Chapter 57

British Association for Parenteral and Enteral Nutrition (2018). 'MUST' calculator. https://www.bapen.org.uk/screening-and-must/must-calculator. Last accessed August 2020.

Fazel, S. and Wolf, A. (2018). Selecting a risk assessment tool to use in practice: A 10-point guide. *Evidence Based Mental Health*. http://ebmh.bmj.com/content/ebmental/21/2/41.full.pdf http://dx.doi.org/10.1136/eb-2017-102861.

Royal College of Physicians (2017). National Early Warning Score 2. https://www.rcplondon.ac.uk/projects/outputs/national-early-warning-score-news-2. Last accessed August 2020.

Chapter 58

Butler, Z.A. (2020). Implementing the National Early Warning Score 2 into pre-registration nurse education. Nursing Standard. doi: 10.7748/ns.2020.e11470.

NHS England (2018). National Early Warning Score (NEWS). https://www.england.nhs.uk/nationalearlywarningscore/#which-patient-groups-should-not-use-news. Last accessed August 2020.

Royal College of Physicians (2017). National Early Warning Score 2. https://www.rcplondon.ac.uk/projects/outputs/national-early-warning-score-news-2. Last accessed August 2020.

Chapter 59

Boreneo, A. (2019). *Standing up for Patient and Public Safety*. Royal College of Nursing: London.

Woodward, S. (2020). *Implementing Patient Safety: Addressing Culture and Values to Help People Work Safely*. Routledge: Oxford.

World Health Organization (2014). Working paper. Preliminary version of minimal information model for patient safety. https://www.who.int/patientsafety/implementation/IMPS_working-paper.pdf?ua=1. Last accessed August 2020.

Chapter 60

Aiken, L.H., Sloane, D.M., Bruyneel, L. et al. (2014). Nurse staffing and education and hospital mortality in nine European countries: A retrospective observational study. *Lancet* 383: 1824–1830.

Griffiths, P., Ball, J., Bloor, K. et al. (2018). Nurse staffing levels, missed vital signs and mortality in hospitals: Retrospective longitudinal observational study. *Health Services and Delivery Research* Vol 38. https://doi.org/10.3310/hsdr06380

Nursing and Midwifery Council (2016). NMC briefing. Appropriate staffing in health and care settings. What is the NMC's interest in staffing? https://www.nmc.org.uk/globalassets/sitedocuments/press/safe-staffing-position-statement.pdf. Last accessed August 2020.

Chapter 61

Nursing and Midwifery Council (NMC) (2019a). Revalidation. https://www.nmc.org.uk/globalassets/sitedocuments/revalidation/how-to-revalidate-booklet.pdf. Last accessed August 2020.

NMC (2019b). Support to help you revalidate. https://www.nmc.org.uk/globalassets/sitedocuments/revalidation/support-to-help-you-revalidate.pdf. Last accessed August 2020.

Royal College of Nursing (2020). Revalidation. https://www.rcn.org.uk/professional-development/revalidation. Last accessed August 2020.

Chapter 62

Mealer, M. (2020). *Coping with Caring: A Nurses' Guide to Better Health and Job Satisfaction*. Taylor and Francis: Abingdon.

NHS (2019). Workforce stress and the supportive organisation. https://www.hee.nhs.uk/sites/default/files/documents/Workforce%20Stress%20and%20the%20Supportive%20Organisation_0.pdf. Last accessed August 2020.

Royal College of Nursing (2016). Resilience. https://rcni.com/hosted-content/rcn/mnd/resilience. Last accessed August 2020.

Chapter 63

NHS Improving Quality (2014). Integrated care and Support Pioneers Programme. Building collaborative teams: A workshop guide for service managers and facilitators. Bringing teams together to deliver joined up care for people who use care and support services. https://www.england.nhs.uk/improvement-hub/wp-content/uploads/sites/44/2019/01/Building-Collaborative-Teams-workshop-guide-2014-1.pdf. Last accessed August 2020.

Royal College of Physicians (2017). Improving teams in healthcare. Resource1: Building effective teams. https://www.rcem.ac.uk//docs/External%20Guidance/ITIH%20R1%20Final.pdf. Last accessed August 2020.

The Health Foundation (2020). How far will integrated health and care systems go in preventing disease? https://www.health.org.uk/news-and-comment/blogs/how-far-will-integrated-health-and-care-systems-go-in-preventing-disease. Last accessed August 2020.

Chapter 64

Department of Health (2012). *Long Term Conditions Compendium of Information*, 3rd Ed. https://assets.publishing.service.gov.uk/government/uploads/system/uploads/attachment_data/file/216528/dh_134486.pdf. Last accessed August 2020.

Naylor, C., Parsonage, M., McDaid, D. et al. (2012). Long-term conditions and mental health the cost of co-morbidities. https://www.kingsfund.org.uk/sites/default/files/field/field_publication_file/long-term-conditions-mental-health-cost-comorbidities-naylor-feb12.pdf. Last accessed August 2020.

Nicol, J and Hollowood, L. (2019). *Nursing Adults with Long Term Conditions*, 3rd Ed. Learning Matters: London.

Chapter 65

Irvine, A. (2019). Immediate care: A stepping stone from hospital to community. *Nursing Older People*. https://rcni.com/nursing-older-people/features/intermediate-care-a-stepping-stone-hospital-to-community-145616. Last accessed August 2020.

NHS Benchmarking Network (2017). Nation audit of intermediate care. Summary report – England. https://s3.eu-west-2.amazonaws.com/nhsbn-static/NAIC+(Providers)/2017/NAIC+England+Summary+Report+-+upload+2.pdf. Last accessed August 2020.

National Institute of Health and Care Excellence (2020). Promoting independence through intermediate care. https://www.nice.org.uk/about/nice-communities/social-care/quick-guides-for-social-care/promoting-independence-through-intermediate-care. Last accessed August 2020.

Chapter 66

National Institute for Health and Care Excellence (2015). Transition between inpatient hospital settings and community or care home settings for adults with social care needs. https://www.nice.org.uk/guidance/ng27/resources/transition-between-inpatient-hospital-settings-and-community-or-care-home-settings-for-adults-with-social-care-needs-pdf-1837336935877. Last accessed August 2020.

Parliamentary and Health Service Ombudsman (2016). A report of investigations into unsafe discharge from hospital. https://www.ombudsman.org.uk/sites/default/files/page/A%20report%20of%20investigations%20into%20unsafe%20discharge%20from%20hospital.pdf. Last accessed August 2020.

Hennessy, S., Nash, M. and Donohue, G. (2020). Enhancing physical health monitoring in people with severe mental illness: The development of a health passport. *Mental Health Practice*. doi: 10.7748/mhp.2020.e1368

Care Quality Commission (2018). Beyond barriers. How older people move between health and social care in England. https://www.cqc.org.uk/sites/default/files/20180702_beyond_barriers.pdf. Last accessed August 2020.

NHS (2015). NHS constitution the NHS belongs to us all. https://assets.publishing.service.gov.uk/government/uploads/system/ uploads/attachment data/file/480482/NHS_Constitution_WEB.pdf. Last accessed August 2020.

Richard, L., Furler, J., Densley, K. et al. (2016). Equity of access to primary healthcare for vulnerable populations: The IMPACT international online survey of innovations. *International Journal for Equity in Health* 64(15). https://doi.org/10.1186/s12939-016-0351-7

Index

Note: Page locators in **bold** indicate tables/boxes. Page locators in *italics* indicate figures. This index uses letter-by-letter alphabetization.

The Nursing Associate at a Glance, First Edition. Ian Peate.
© 2021 John Wiley & Sons Ltd. Published 2021 by John Wiley & Sons Ltd.